TONGUE CANCER AND I

TONGUE CANCER AND I

BY

DEV R MADHAVAN

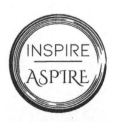

Published in 2021 in Great Britain by Inspire *Aspire* Publishing

Copyright © 2021 Dev R Madhavan
Cover and formatting by The Amethyst Angel

ISBN: 978-1-9999618-0-0

Any web addresses or links mentioned may have changed since publication.

Disclaimer

The author of this book does not dispense medical advice or prescribe the use of any technique as a form of treatment for physical, emotional or medical problem. This book is not intended to be a substitute for individual diagnosis and treatment by a qualified medical professional, who will make recommendations for treatment based upon each reader's medical history and current medical condition. The intent of the author is to share their own experience, and to offer general information to help you in your quest for wellbeing. In the event you use any of the information in this book for yourself, the author and publisher assume no responsibility for your actions or the consequences of those actions.

Exclusions

Tracheostomy and Chemotherapy are not covered in this book as the author did not undergo this type of surgery or treatment

Dedicated to my parents, brothers and immediate family; thank you for all your love and support.

To the reader; may this book inspire and enlighten you to have the courage and hope to overcome your challenges and pursue your dreams.

CONTENTS

It was Tuesday 6th September 2016.

I was at the West Middlesex University Hospital, for a biopsy result. As I entered the room to meet the doctor, I took a silent deep breath. I tried to be calm and objective.

Doctor: 'We have your biopsy results and I'm afraid it's not good news. You have Squamous cell carcinoma.'

The news hit me like a sledgehammer.

I had cancer.

Little did I know, that what felt like the end of the world, would be the beginning of an epic journey.

INTRODUCTION

The journey from a diagnosis of tongue cancer to complete recovery is not an easy one. I certainly found it difficult, and have had to endure and overcome many challenges along the way. For those of you who have just been diagnosed with tongue cancer, or are currently in the middle of being treated for it, this book is for you. I have documented my journey, including the different feelings that I experienced, the medical treatment I received, and the stages that I went through in recovering from this illness. Not only do I want this book to be a source of emotional support, but I also want to keep you informed, and prepare you for the events and treatments that may be ahead of you.

For those that have recovered from tongue cancer, you may also find some great insights in the chapters on Treatments to Aid Recovery and Life After Cancer.

To the family and friends of someone with tongue cancer, I

also wanted to keep you informed about what your loved one will be going through. This will help you to have a much better understanding of what they are experiencing, and how you can support, care and help them through their journey.

And finally to all other readers, may you find some nuggets of gold which may help you to appreciate and understand what is important in your life and how to live a life more fulfilled.

In the following pages, you will also find practical recommendations, key learning & action points and observations. I share what helped me to stay strong, and what encouraged and motivated me, during the tough times. I hope you will also find them beneficial.

In Appendix A and B, I have provided my timelines of events, both in hospital and after hospital. This will give you a bigger picture of things, before diving into the detail.

I sincerely hope that the content of this book inspires and empowers you to overcome tongue cancer, and that may it serve and inform you in a positive light. By having a clearer picture of the events and challenges ahead of you, I am confident that you will be better prepared to overcome and succeed.

CHAPTER 1
BEFORE THE DIAGNOSIS

My closest friends would describe my personality as happy, smiley, friendly and sociable. I'm someone who always looks at life in a positive and optimistic way. I always have a smile on my face, even if I may not be feeling that great inside. I also consider myself to be quite driven, to the extent where I will often push myself a little too far to succeed. I would not describe this as egotistical, because my ambitions are not achieved at the cost of others, but it's more about overtly putting pressure on myself and over doing it.

I was 44 years old and I had a healthy outlook on life. I did not smoke and would only drink alcohol, socially, once a week. I kept active, going to the gym, doing weights, resistance training and cardio exercise. I also played tennis twice a week. My close friends also had a healthy outlook on life, and we would always be sharing training tips and new exercises to try, and would help one another improve.

In short – life was pretty good. I was living at home with my family, had a great, well-paid job, and was on the cusp of purchasing a second property, in which I would live. In my free time, I enjoyed playing tennis, catching up with friends and family, dining out, going to the cinema, attending parties and taking lots of holidays. Brazil, Thailand and Ibiza provided me with some of my favourite memories. I was also attending personal development and transformation seminars and workshops, as I had a passion for learning and growing and improving myself.

One of my favourite events is, Unleash the Power Within, by Tony Robbins. I've attended this event a couple of times, both as a participant and as part of the volunteer event crew. It is a very entertaining learning experience, with over 6,000 people from around the world in attendance. The event is a great way to create forward momentum in your life. Overall, I was living quite a fast-paced life, and while that did feel good, it also came with some pressures.

Early in 2016, I was handed a new project management role at my company. It was a more senior role, which brought more responsibility and opportunity. I rose to the challenge, working extremely hard and pushing myself, while supporting and molding the team, processes and procedures, until we were a finely tuned unit capable of efficiently executing the delivery of projects, from start to finish.

I had spent the past 20 years prior to this role carving out a professional career, working my way up the corporate ladder, and this promotion felt like a reward. I was on the right path, and I was prepared to work myself into the ground to move forwards. The problem was, I had not stopped to ask myself if this was really me. I had simply assumed that I was doing the right thing, and suddenly I found that I was focusing far too much on work. Despite managing the project efficiently I was not managing the stress it created effectively. I started to neglect other key areas of my life, such as playing tennis and being socially active with friends, which led to a poor work/life balance. With the added pressure that I placed on myself, it was inevitable there would be an impact on my health.

In addition to this, there were also a series of family bereavements that had sadly occurred, over the course of 4 years, which also added to the emotional pressures of life.

I'd definitely recommend taking stock of your own work/life balance and the emotional pressures that you may have, and give careful consideration to how they might be impacting your health. Sometimes we can get so busy, operating on autopilot, that we don't stop, take a pause, assess our lives and make changes to serve our health and wellbeing.

CHAPTER 2
DIAGNOSIS

THE WHITE CLOUD

In April 2016 I noticed a white blemish on the left side of my tongue. I was not sure what it was, and it seemed very harmless. I tried brushing it hard with my toothbrush, and also used a tongue scraper to see if it would come off, but to no avail. Sometimes I did this a bit too hard and it would bleed. After a few days, I decided to leave it and let nature take its course. It still amazes me that I did this. You will often hear dentists remark on how people will go to the doctors right away if their leg continually bleeds, but when their gums bleed they simply chalk it off to rough brushing, or simply ignore it altogether. I used to think that this was just a cliché, but now I understand it. In my case, I was quite confident that the white cloud would eventually disappear from my tongue. Besides, I was too busy focusing on my career to worry about it. It would go away, I was sure of it.

Make sure you see your dentist every 6 months - they might spot something that you do not. Even if you don't like going to the dentist, I recommend going and asking the dentist to be very, very gentle. If they are not, then change your dentist until you find one that suits you.

On top of this, I was also not one for seeing the dentist. I think most people hate going to the dentist, but at that time it had been over a year since I'd been. I often found that they were very rough with my teeth and gums, and as a result, I wasn't keen on making an appointment. So, I waited. It was only in retrospect I realized that this was a big mistake.

SEEING THE DOCTOR

In early August 2016, after returning from a lovely holiday in Bodrum, I had noticed that the white cloud had now turned into a lump, just smaller than a two pence coin. It was now growing and protruding outwards from the left side of my tongue. I decided to see my GP, and when the GP analysed it, she immediately advised that I get it checked out at West Middlesex University Hospital, at the Oral and Maxillofacial Clinic, where they would perform a biopsy.

I felt a bit better that some form of action was being taken to investigate what this lump was. The GP did not say what she thought it was, and I didn't ask for her opinion, feeling that it was better to wait for the biopsy results.

During the month of August, my dad was in hospital having a triple heart bypass. My thoughts and time were spent with my dad and family, and visiting the hospital regularly. I spared little thought for my own health. Once my dad was back home resting and recovering, I advised the family that I had an issue with my tongue and that I need to go for a biopsy. They were calm and agreed that we should take things one step at a time, before speculating what it could be.

BIOPSY

On the 30th August 2016 I had the biopsy. I had not had a biopsy before, so didn't know what to expect. What I did know was that I had to get it done. My mindset was focused, and I understood clearly that whatever the procedure was, it was going to help me.

The nurses were very kind and gentle and asked me to sit in a reclining 'dental' chair. The nurse had a large syringe with quite a long needle, which she injected into the left side of my mouth. This was to make my mouth numb. It was not painful, maybe a slight prick. It took 5 to 10 minutes for the anaesthetic to take effect. The nurse then proceeded to take a biopsy. They used a laser instrument to slice off a part of the 'two pence coin' lump, on the left-hand side of my tongue. I did not feel anything, which was great. The hospital advised that the results should take about 1 week, and prescribed me with "Difflam" mouthwash. This helps to cool and numb the mouth. I was also advised to take some painkillers, paracetamol, as the tongue would feel very sore, and to also be careful when eating over the next few days.

Over the next 3 to 5 days, my mouth was indeed very sore. I used the Difflam mouthwash regularly, to manage the pain and discomfort and to help ease things when eating. It had a nice cooling sensation, which had a calming effect on my mouth.

DIAGNOSIS

It was Tuesday 6th September 2016.

I was at the West Middlesex University Hospital, for a biopsy result. As I entered the room to meet the doctor, I took a silent deep breath. I tried to be calm and objective.

Doctor: 'We have your biopsy results and I'm afraid it's not good news. You have Squamous cell carcinoma, stage 2.'

The news hit me like a sledgehammer.

I had cancer.

In that moment I received the diagnosis, lots of things were going through my mind. "I have Stage 2 Tongue Cancer. Is this actually happening? Wow! Is the life I had slipping away?" Then I got a grip of myself. I reminded myself that I was here, I was alive. I focused on being present and objective, on how I could overcome this. Suddenly, my career which had been my sole focus, was no longer the priority.

Survival mode kicked in, and I felt like I was in a Rocky movie, accepting the challenge and having to bounce back from adversity. Except that my opponent were rogue cells in my body, not another human being. I had to acknowledge that this was my situation, whether I liked it or not, and that I had to be strong for my parents and brothers, to give myself the best chance to beat this. My mum was in the room with me, and she did not take the diagnosis well at all. It was hard, as we had just lost my aunt (my mum's sister) to cancer the year before. So this was hitting very close to home. I embraced my mum, and tried to console her. It's not easy for any mum to have her child go through this, I knew I needed to be strong for her.

The doctor explained the next steps to me. An MRI and CT Scan would be scheduled, to understand the location and depth of the cancer, and then a medical team would determine a plan of action, beginning with major surgery. It was indeed a lot to take in. I took a deep breath in, and thanked the doctor for his support and kindness.

Following the diagnosis, mum and I went home, and I told my other family members. They took some time to digest the news. They were very objective and supportive, and needed time to process the information. It is strangely funny how life can change so quickly. How fragile it can become.

The things I thought were so important, became meaningless and I wished that I could just go back in time, to when it was just a white cloud, five months before, and got it diagnosed then; as I am sure any surgery at that point would have been less invasive. Whilst I couldn't help feeling upset, nevertheless, I knew I had to release these feelings and focus on the next steps.

I made the decision to write a concise Facebook message, to a select group of friends across different social circles, to briefly explain what was happening. I did this because I did not want cancer to own me and I wanted to take some form of positive action and expression, and to convey to them not to worry. I wrote that I planned to overcome it, and for them to cherish their health and make the most out of their life – as no one knows when a challenge will come around. This declaration empowered me, gave me a sense of control, and made me feel better that it was now out in the open.

I received lots of lovely messages of support and care, which was really nice to have. A few of my close friends wanted to meet up, before the major surgery, which I accepted and was very happy about.

CHAPTER 3
AFTER THE DIAGNOSIS

ACCEPTANCE

When hit with news of an illness like cancer, coming to terms with where you are can be very difficult to accept. Lots of thoughts might be running through your head. Why me? How did this happen? If I had done this or that, then perhaps this would not have happened. My thoughts were: "I can't believe it! Is this really happening? Is my life going to be cut short, or diminished in some capacity?"

It's okay to go through this questioning stage. It's completely natural, and I like to think that it was part of the healing process. When I asked these questions, and allowed myself to feel the range of emotions, it helped me to fully express and clarify my thoughts, and it put me in a better state of mind. As they say, it is better out than in.

The uncertainty of what's to come can also be scary and overwhelming. I found that once I processed my thoughts and feelings and accepted where I was, I felt better. I made the decision to focus on one day at a time. One step of the plan at a time. Focusing on what I needed to do each day in terms of treatments and routines seemed to lessen the load, and made things easier to manage. Trying to consider the bigger picture was too overwhelming, especially when the outcome was unknown. So I just focused on the tasks in front of me, and took each day at a time.

 Can you look at where you are, and accept it? It is only possible to change the things we can accept, so acceptance of your current situation is the very first step towards healing.

NEXT STEPS

Whilst waiting to have the MRI and CT scans, I started to look at ways in which I could get myself into a better place of positivity and progress. I already had quite a healthy diet, I exercised regularly, and had family support, so I did the following:

QUIT CAFFIENE

I knew that I had to get my body, mind and soul as calm as possible. I made the decision right then, as soon as I was diagnosed, to stop drinking coffee or any caffeinated drinks. I felt that these prevented me from being in a calm state. I was a regular coffee drinker, having at least 1-2 cups daily, mostly because I loved the taste. Despite the daily habit, I stopped drinking coffee with amazing ease. It is unbelievable what you can do when you focus. I stopped it entirely, cold turkey, because I really wanted to be in a calm and relaxed physical and mental state. I had no reasons to have a 'get up and go' or 'get things done' attitude, which I associate with coffee. I soon realized that I could still do a lot and be in a calmer state, without caffeine.

MEDITATION

I also quickly turned to meditation. Again, I was thinking about how I could get myself into a calm and relaxed state, and how could I control my breathing. So, I went online and bought the book, *Mindfulness; a practical guide to finding peace in a frantic world*. I had heard about this book from someone, and the summary content sounded spot on. The book came with a CD of meditations, and it played a major part in getting me through the treatments. Every day, I performed the "body scan" meditation. It really helped to keep me in a peaceful state.

JOURNALING

I bought a number of notebooks, which I used for journaling. I found that documenting my daily thoughts, affirmations, the things I was looking forward to and many other topics, helped me to process things and provided some self-healing. I had not journaled before, so this was new to me. This was another form of self-expression which was very therapeutic and helped me to channel my thoughts onto the page, keeping my mind free of any negative noise.

AFFIRMATIONS

I then focused on my daily thoughts and language. I wanted to instill in myself the belief that I was going to get better, and to be as strong and resilient as possible. I did this by writing out my own affirmations in my journal.

These were as follows:

- I AM Positive, Strong and Calm.

- I CAN Beat this.

- I WILL Beat this.

- I AM Beating this.

- It's ONLY Stage 1 and is only on my tongue (I said this rather than Stage 2 as I wanted to build the thought that it was less serious than it was).

- I WILL make a 100% Recovery.

- I AM making a 100% Recovery.

- Stay Focused!

- This Operation Serves Me! It will help me to be healthy again and have a second chance at life.

Every day I would read these affirmations and imprint them in my mind, heart and soul. I would use these words in all of my conversations, be it verbal or written, with friends and family. I would live and breathe these.

I eventually produced my own longer affirmation that I used throughout my journey and still do to this day. It is as follows:

"I am Positive and Strong, Calm and Relaxed. My life is filled with Love, Joy and Happiness and my life is filled with Abundance."

 WRITE YOUR OWN AFFIRMATIONS

If you can produce your own affirmations that really resonate with you, the effect can be amazing. Use them every day, breathe them in and believe them.

VISIONS FOR THE FUTURE

I thought about all the wonderful things I wanted to see and do in the future after having a successful operation and recovery. I wrote them all down, and then visualised where I wanted to be – I mean I could really see it! My list looked like this:

- I will see my 6-year-old niece graduate from university.

- I will take Mum to the U.S Open Tennis Championships next year (2017)

- I will help others who are about to go or are going through oral cancer.

- I will have a simpler life, less technology based.

- I will settle down, with an amazing soul of a woman, and raise a family

- I will see my younger brother settle down.

- I will choose a restaurant that Dad likes. (This was an amusing, ongoing thing, where the last place I chose for the family to eat, was very bad).

- I will meet my friends for lunch at Tibits (one of my favourite vegetarian restaurants. Not that I was a vegetarian, but I really liked the food and ambience.)

I am happy to say that I managed to achieve some of these. For example, Mum and I did go to New York and watch the 2017 U.S Open Tennis Championships and the family have indeed been to some great restaurants.

Write out your visions - the things that really mean a lot to you. Things you want to do, see, have, experience. Draw them, collect photos of them, create a vision diary or board or a list like I did. Close your eyes and see them taking shape. They will give you something positive to focus on.

ACTIVITIES I WANT TO DO

I made a list of activities that I wanted to do post-operation/post-recovery.

- I want to play more tennis and improve my game. (Tennis is my favourite sport and I've had a love for this game for many years)

- I want to take up dance again – salsa, ballroom, tap, street dance, as it's lots of fun.

- Do more local nature-based activities – walks in the park, hikes.

- I would love to continue doing my exciting travel adventures around the world. There's so much to see.

- I would like to go to more comedy shows, theatre, concerts and events

- I would like to learn and do more meditation

- I will learn more about mentorship and coaching and help develop and support others

- I would love to do a skydive, even though heights are not my favourite thing.

I did actually play more tennis, took up Lindy Hop dancing, did more meditation and travelled to so many wonderful places.

What activities do you want to do after your successful operation and recovery?

Write these down, draw them, and picture them in your mind.

GOING ON LONG-TERM SICK LEAVE

During the second week of September 2016, I went on long-term sick leave. My line manager and company were really supportive and understood that I needed to be in a less stressful state and be focused only on getting better. It was vital for me to rest and take things easy. If you can do the same, I highly recommend this. You need to stay focused on your health and prepare yourself for the challenges ahead. I found the Macmillan Cancer Support Guide Books called, *Understanding Head And Neck Cancers* and *Work and Cancer*, very useful. These books explained what Employments rights, financial help and benefits I could seek.

If sick leave is not an option, see if you can reduce your hours, and work with your employer to create a better balance. Look into what benefits might be available, if finances are an issue. Dealing with these things early on means not having to worry about them while you are undergoing treatment, when all your focus needs to be on healing and resting.

IMPLEMENT DAILY ROUTINES

I decided to implement a daily routine. I would get up at the same time each morning, make my bed, have a shower, brush my teeth, have a warm lemon drink, and then breakfast. I wanted to start every day on the right foot. I also needed to keep myself occupied, now that I wasn't at work. I didn't want to sit still and think about things, but I also didn't want to be overly busy, because my body needed time to rest. I really encourage you to create a daily routine, and not just when you are facing illness. It really helps to create a balance and to allow you time to destress and relax. There were times when I would go for a walk in the park, or go to the gym for a very light workout, or even go to a local museum. I found that as long as I was fairly active, I felt more positive.

WHY DID I GET IT?

I spent time reviewing and reflecting on why this was happening to me. I would consider myself a rational person who looks at things logically. I read lots of books throughout my journey, I was thirsty for knowledge and answers and more peace of mind. I did my research and if you are where I was, I also encourage you to do so as well. Reflecting on the possible causes is not so you can blame yourself. It's not so that you can regret your past behaviours, or berate yourself for your diet or your life choices. Doing this reflection and understanding the possible causes of developing cancer is about empowerment. It's about understanding your body, the effect your choices have on your body, and how you have the power to change those choices.

TOP 3 REASONS

The top 3 reasons for getting Tongue Cancer are as follows: [source: my doctors]

1. Smoking

2. Drinking Alcohol

3. Getting the Human Papilloma Virus (HPV)

I had socially smoked in the past, maybe 15 to 20 years previously, but that was only 1-2 cigarettes, once a week. I did tend to have 1 or 2 vodka tonics every time I went out socially, which was a maximum of 2 nights per week.

With HPV, you tend to get this from sexual contact, be it oral or vaginal intercourse, protected or unprotected. I got tested for this and there was no detection of this virus orally or on the genitals.

So, why did I get tongue cancer? I wasn't a prime candidate for it. The doctors stated that it was "just my bad luck". I appreciated their viewpoint, but I knew there was always a reason why things happened, even if you didn't know exactly why.

I chose to look within myself, and came up with my own list of possible reasons. Some of them I am sure would not make sense to others, but to me they did.

MY REASONS

A) Immune System

I felt that perhaps my immune system was just not strong enough to fight off the cancer, which perhaps had been dormant in my system. I hardly get colds and flu, but I'd had skin rashes in the past, which generally flared up when I was work-stressed and run down. The year before the diagnosis had been a stressful year for me – working in a new, more challenging role – and I had pushed myself really hard. I strongly believe that this played a part in making me more prone to illness.

B) Forgiveness

Bearing grudges is never healthy. I read a book called *Forgive for Good* by Dr. Fred Luskin. One of the key things I took from this book is that holding onto grudges can cross over from your emotional to your physical state. This hit home for me, as I did have a number of past family, friends, work colleagues and acquaintances whom I had not forgiven for various things.

During my recovery at home, I practiced forgiving each of these people. It really helped with my peace of mind. I also looked within, for things that I had not forgiven myself for. I realised that I was too hard on myself, and needed to shift my perspective and accept that it is okay not to achieve everything and do everything. I believe that forgiving yourself for your past choices and behaviour is very powerful and healing.

C) My focus

After a little reflection, I realised that I focused too much on things that I did not have yet, and put too much pressure on myself to get these. For example, I had not purchased my own UK property yet, and I had not settled down and had kids. My thoughts were often of lack, of what I did not have, and I had become far too fixated on obtaining things. I adapted my thinking and affirmed that it was more than okay to not have these. Time to focus on what I did have! I have wonderful parents, brothers and family. I have a safe and secure roof over my head. I have food and water and I can make my own decisions, and I have a great job. I began to write in my journal what I was grateful for, and who and what I appreciated in my life.

What are you grateful for in your life? Have you expressed that gratitude? Why not write a list in your journal or write a thank you card to someone who has supported you?

CHAPTER 4
BEFORE THE OPERATION

WHAT DID THE TUMOUR LOOK LIKE?

I wanted to share with you what my tumour looked like. It's important for you to really comprehend what it looked like, as I know this will help you see how it can grow, if it is not identified and addressed in an earlier stage.

By the time of diagnosis, the tumour had grown into a circular lump the size of a two pence coin. It was on the left lateral side of my tongue, and was growing in all directions, protruding outwards towards my teeth.

On the next pages are some pictures of what it looked like, one week before my operation.

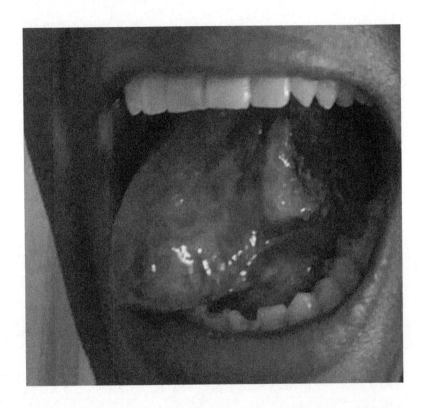

Picture 1

This picture gives you some perspective of the size of the tumour against the whole tongue.

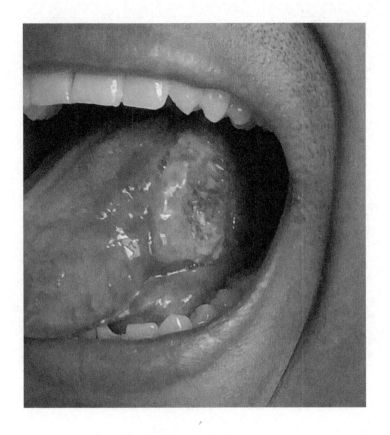

Picture 2

This is a closer look at the tumour. You can see the clearly defined circular shape. The centre is slightly darker, as this would bleed sometimes when it rubbed against my teeth.

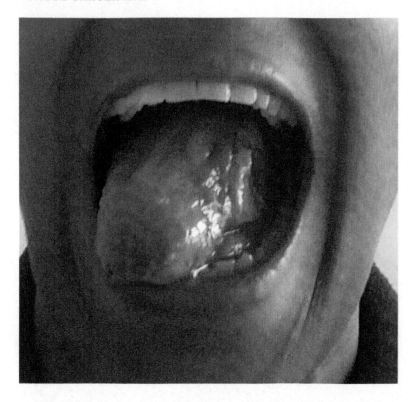

Picture 3

In this picture you can see how the tumour was growing outwards and encroaching on my teeth. At this point, it impeded my speech and I was finding it difficult to pronounce some words, and sounded like I had a lisp. I knew the tumour was quickly getting worse, but I had to remain focused on the next positive step. On the bright side, I do have nice teeth!

Cancer is a mutation of cells that grow out of control. Which you can definitely see in the pictures, in how 'alien' it looks. By the day of the operation, it had grown a lot more, but I

28

didn't take any more photos. By that point, I knew I had no choice, I had to have the operation, to give me the best chance of recovering.

MRI AND CT SCANS

Within one week of diagnosis I had the CT scan (September 10th 2016) and MRI scan (September 13th 2016). I really appreciate the NHS and doctors fast tracking this process, I have no doubt that it improved my odds considerably.

Having the MRI scan was a very interesting experience. The doctors advised that I would be in the chamber for a duration between 15 to 30 minutes. I had heard stories from others that the chamber could be quite tight and claustrophobic, but I did not let that phase me. Using my meditation practices and slow breathing techniques, I remained extremely calm. I would highly recommend practicing such techniques prior to having the MRI.

The process of having the MRI was as follows:

I lay down, on my back, in the chamber. I wore headphones, provided by the hospital, whilst they performed the scan. There were also pads securing my shoulders and neck into place, so that they did not move during the scan.

I knew it was important to remain in a calm and relaxed state, and believe that this procedure was going to help me. When the bed was retracted back into the chamber, I chose to close my eyes and meditate. I thought that watching the bed retract all the way back into the enclosed chamber would make me feel afraid, so to overcome this I shut my eyes, and it worked. Throughout the scan, I kept my eyes closed. This was a personal choice. They do have a looking glass, so if my eyes were open, it reflects out at 90 degrees, so that I could see outside the chamber.

When the MRI scan started, I heard approximately 20 different sorts of sounds in the background, whilst listening to music. I blocked those sounds out and focused on my affirmations and visualisations. I also slowed down my breathing, and kept myself in the most peaceful and relaxed state.

Inside my mind I was chanting, "I am positive and strong, calm and relaxed. My life is filled with love, joy and happiness and abundance". At the same time, I was picturing myself healthy and fit the following year, with family and friends by my side. By slowing down everything and keeping the mind very clear and peaceful, I was able to remain in a zen-like state, for as long as was required.

I found the experience of having the CT scan much easier than the MRI Scan. The nurses injected me with a special contrast dye, which helps to capture good quality images, of the internal structures of my body. This would help identify the location, size and shape of the tumour. When they injected me, I got a warm feeling in the genital and rectal area, as if I was going to pass urine, but that was ok. The CT scan apparatus is circular in shape and only scans part of the body at a time. You feel much more at ease as it does not enclose the whole body.

TUMOUR GROWTH AND THE WAITING GAME

It was not easy to wait for the results of my scans. During this time it felt as if the tumour was growing. This was of great concern to me, because the more it grew, the more of the tongue they would have to cut away. My speech became more impeded by the growth of the tumour. I obviously felt scared and worried, but I realised I could not do anything about it. So, I decided to focus on being positive, saying to myself that it was okay and that the tumour had stopped growing. I stuck to my daily routine, concentrated on what progress I could make that day, in anything that I did. Again, I was just trying to take one day at a time and take my mind off things.

RESULTS OF THE MRI AND CT

On September 22nd 2016, just over a week after having the MRI scan, I met up with doctors to discuss the results, the plan of action, the surgical approach and the date of the operation.

The results from the MRI and CT scans would show the doctors where the cancer was and help them to plan the approach they were going to take for surgery. The great news was that the results showed the cancer was localised and had not spread, and the staging of the cancer was still classed as stage 2. I was so happy when I heard this, and felt so relieved. Inside I was saying, "Yes, I can do this! Yes, I can beat this!" However, there was a caveat – which was that the scanning technology was not 100% accurate – and this also needed to be factored into the surgical approach. They would only know what the extent of the cancer was, once they were in the operating theatre.

MEETING THE DOCTORS

Prior to receiving my scan results, the doctors had a multi-disciplinary team (MDT) meeting with all of the staff working on my case. This meeting comprised the surgeons, Macmillan clinical nurse specialist, anesthetists, speech and language therapists, dieticians and radiologists. They were all there to discuss my case, determine the approach for the operation and provide support throughout my recovery. On the same day as receiving my MRI and CT scan results, I also met up with the team. This was a great experience, as it allowed me the chance to discuss in detail what the operation entailed. Everyone was positive, professional, well organised and really nice. They made me feel at ease and I was just really grateful that they were there for me.

The lead surgeon consultant expressed that the operation would require the left lateral tongue to be treated with a "left partial glossectomy, left neck dissection and reconstruction with a radial forearm free flap, with post-operative radiotherapy and possibly chemotherapy." To break this down in simple terms, the operation would consist of:

- Removing the tumour from the left lateral tongue with clear margins.

- Partial removal of left salivary glands.

- Cutting a layer of skin, above the wrist of the nondominant hand, and also removing one vein from that forearm. Then stitching the skin flap to the gap made on the left lateral tongue and providing this flap with a blood supply by connecting the vein, that was taken from my forearm, to the inside of my throat.

- The layer of skin that was removed from my forearm would then be replaced by cutting a patch of skin from the left-hand side of my tummy. Then stitching this patch of skin above my hand. The area where the vein was removed, was also sewn up.

- A neck dissection on my left-hand side, from my lower left ear down across to the front centre of my neck would be performed. Then they would remove 56 lymph nodes so that they could test for any cancer. The dissection was recommended as the scanning technology was not accurate enough. I agreed to have this, as I wanted peace of mind that the cancer had not spread to my lymph nodes and through to the lymphatic system, as this could lead to secondary cancer appearing in other parts of the body. After the removal of the lymph nodes, I would then be stitched back up.

- During the operation if the airway is affected and it's difficult to breathe then there may need to be a tracheostomy (incision in the windpipe) to aid breathing.

- The operation would require 2 shifts of staff and would

take up to 12 hours to complete.

All of this information was a lot to take in. It was major reconstructive surgery, and I was placing my trust in the medical team to look after me. I also asked myself what choice I had. In my mind, I did not have any other choice, and surgery was definitely the only option for me.

The lead surgeon consultant asked if I had any questions. I did not have any. He then went on to explain what the risks of surgery were and the post-operation side effects.

They were as follows:

- Excess mouth secretions directly after the operation.

- Dry mouth – due to partial left salivary glands being removed.

- Possible loss of speech.

- Partial loss of nerve muscle on the left-hand side of mouth.

- Loss of feeling on left-hand side of face and ear.

- Droopiness of left-hand side of face

- Difficulty in swallowing

- Intravenous lines and drains will be attached.

- A nasogastric (NG) tube will be fed through the nose into the stomach for feeding.

I am sure there were a few more risks and side effects, which you can read about in the Macmillian Cancer Support Head and Neck Cancer Guide. I accepted all of these, as again I felt that surgery was my only option.

The doctors then advised that they would like to perform the operation on Friday 30th September 2016. I was so happy, as this was only a week away. My concern was that the tumour was growing, and the more it grew the more tongue they would have to cut away, making it less likely that I would be able to speak. So, I was over the moon when they said it would be in a week's time. This gave me so much hope.

Depending on your situation, if you can avoid having the tracheostomy then I would highly recommend this. When I was in the ward, after surgery, I saw a lot of patients with "trachees". They were unable to talk and the windpipe hole that was made required regular cleaning and maintaining. I could see that these patients were in a lot more discomfort than myself – since I hadn't had one. You may not have a choice in this, but if you can ask your surgeon to do their best to avoid giving you a "trachee", then do it.

The second recommendation I have is this: if you can avoid having the neck dissection that would great. Whilst the doctors stitch you up really well, the scarring along the neck leaves a tightness, which can remain for a long time. Five years after my surgery I still have this, although I have learnt to live with it. This tightness can also cause partial difficulty in swallowing. Again, depending on your journey and what your doctor advises, you might not have this choice, but I felt it was important to inform you of the post-recovery problems you might experience.

THE PRE-OPERATIVE ASSESSMENT TESTS

Before the operation I needed to have some tests, to assess whether I was fit to go ahead with it. This was called the pre-op assessment, and I had this on the 23rd September 2016. The test took approximately 3 hours and included the following:

- Blood tests.

- Weight and height taken.

- Documenting any medical allergies.

The tests went well and there were no issues.

I also met up with the speech and language therapists, and also the dietician. They discussed what to expect after surgery. This included not being able to speak immediately, whilst my mouth was healing. We also discussed if I had any food allergies, and that I would be fed through a NG tube, for a period of time, whilst my mouth healed.

The nurses also provided me with an information sheet, with details of what to do the day before the operation. One of the key points was not to eat anything at least 12 hours before surgery, so as to avoid any vomiting under anaesthetic.

FAMILY AND FRIENDS MEETUP

Before my operation there were two occasions that really boosted my spirits. My 6-year-old niece gave me a surprise visit, which made me so happy. It gave me an inner strength and focus, to get better so that I could be there for her and see her grow up. I also had a number of close friends come to see me. They were all very supportive and made me laugh and smile.

I would highly recommend meeting up with those who are important in your life. It helps make you stronger to get through the surgery, and keeps you in positive spirits prior to the big event.

CHAPTER 5
PREPARING FOR
THE OPERATION

During the weeks between the diagnosis and the day of the operation, I began to prepare myself. I concentrated on what activities I could do so that I was fully prepared for the operation, my stay in hospital, and up to when I was discharged from hospital. I looked at what I could control and what could help me.

KEY ACTIONS

• I bought an A5 writing pad and pens so that I could journal my thoughts and record events.

• I bought a number of thank you cards, so that when I was discharged I could write to all the doctors and nurses and say thank you.

• I had a haircut, shaved, and cut my nails before going to hospital.

• I arranged to meet up with friends two weeks before the operation.

• I advised my immediate family that I did not want any friends visiting me during the hospital stay. This was so that I could remain clear and focused on recovering.

• I nominated one of my best friends to be my spokesperson. My family would contact him with progress updates, which could then be communicated to my social circle. This made life a lot easier for me and my family, so that we did not have to worry about too many communications to others, and we could manage our energy carefully.

From the above, you can see the project manager in me. I was planning ahead and trying to be prepared, as much as possible.

BAG PREPARATION

I was advised that I would be staying in hospital for up to two weeks, and would be required to take a bag containing my belongings. I would recommend that you prepare two bags.

SMALLER BAG

I prepared a small bag, which I would need directly after the operation, when I was moved to the recovery ward. Hopefully the contents of my bag will help you to pack your own:

• A pair of slippers – you will need these to walk around for the next day or so, and it's best to keep your feet warm, as the hospital floor is cold.

• Lip balm - Lip balm is very useful, as your lips will be very dry after surgery. The nurses do provide "lanolin" but I preferred a normal lip balm.

• Eye Mask – These are very useful, as I found that the recovery ward had lights that were very bright and penetrating. I recommend getting an eye mask that has an elastic backing rather than Velcro connections, as it will be easier to put this on using the hand that's not been operated on, or alternatively ask a nurse to help.

• Ear plugs/headphones – I did not pack any, but in hindsight I think it would have helped, to block out noise from the ward, and to help keep calm.

• Fully charged mobile phone and charger – I did not use these but worth having as a safety net.

OPTIONAL:

• A small pocket-sized book, called the Zohar. It's a spiritual text, which was given to me by a good friend. I am not religious but I really appreciated the gift and took this with me for enriched support. I would recommend having a book that inspires you.

MEDIUM-SIZED BAG

I prepared a medium-sized sports bag for when I was moved to the general ward. My family could then bring this bag to me when required. In the bag, I had packed the following contents:

• Dressing gown.

- Pyjamas.

- Reading books.

- My A5 writing pad and pens.

- Thank you cards.

- Headphones.

- Ear plugs.

- Massage ball.

- Socks and underwear – only needed for the last few days before being discharged.

- Other clothes: t-shirt, jeans, fleece, scarf.

- Trainers.

- Toiletry bag and contents – including cotton swabs and a flannel to clean face.

- Shower slippers.

- Small torch and small mirror – this is very useful when you have to clean your mouth after surgery, so that you can see what you are doing.

KEEPING BUSY

In the week before the operation, I was extremely worried about the growth of the tumour and was eager to get it removed. Each day, I tried keeping myself busy so as not to think about things too much. I would do the following:

• Watch funny movies and TV shows. For example, I love watching Impractical Jokers. This made me laugh and put me in good spirits.

• I would also go to the cinema – this kept me busy and got me out of the house.

• I practiced meditation, every day, which comprised listening to a guided 10-minute meditation on The Body Scan. This really helped to keep me calm and relaxed and helped control my breathing.

• On a daily basis I internally chanted my affirmations with great conviction, and also spent time focusing on a positive outcome to the surgery and all the wonderful visions I had for the future.

• I also developed a large appetite for reading. I was hungry for self-help books, even more so than before. The reading material kept me positive, strong and productive. Some of the books I read are as follows:

o *The Secret* by Rhonda Byrne.

o *The Key to Living the Law of Attraction* by Jack Canfield and D.D Watkins.

o *The Art of Happiness* by HH Dalai Lama & Howard C. Cutler.

o *Aspire* by Kevin Hall.

All of these books carried inspiring messages, which helped me to maintain a positive mindset. If you can find books that will help you, give it a go. It will take your mind off things for a while.

ENJOY YOUR FAVOURITE FOODS

In retrospect, I wish I had also indulged in my favourite foods before the operation, and I highly recommend that you embrace and enjoy all the foods you love to eat prior to the operation, if you are at that point yourself. Unfortunately, I did not do this. For 8 to 10 weeks after the operation, you may not be able to eat these foods. You may also find that your mouth might become hypersensitive and you can no longer tolerate the foods you used to love. In my case I found that I couldn't eat curries anymore – they were just too spicy. So go ahead and eat the pizza, the curries and burgers – enjoy them now, as it may be a while before you can indulge in these foods again!

WRITING IN MY JOURNAL

As I mentioned in the previous chapter, I wrote out the following in my journal:

• On the back pages I made a list of the following:

    o My affirmations.

    o My visions for the future.

    o Activities I want to do once out of hospital.

    o Activities I would love to do once fully recovered.

o A checklist for contents of my bag when I stay in hospital.

Aside from the checklist, every day whilst in hospital, I would review the above, to keep me in good spirits. Concentrating on all the wonderful things that I would do once I fully recovered, made me strong enough to get through things.

• On the front pages I did the following:

o First 5 pages – Automated written responses. After the operation, the mouth needs to heal, and therefore you should not talk, unless the doctors say that it is okay to do so. Therefore, writing out what you need, can really help. For example, writing things like thank you, thank you for your wonderful support, and any questions that you may have for the doctors and nurses.

o Next 10 pages – I left these blank so that I could capture the timeline of events and my progress and journal my thoughts.

YOUR STORY – VICTIM OR HERO?

The story you tell yourself about yourself can really have an impact on you, your self-talk, your thoughts and your outlook on life. The cliché, "Are you the victim or hero of your story?" rings true here.

As part of my preparation, I asked myself who inspired me in terms of overcoming adversity in their lives. My parents definitely came top of the list. They have been very inspiring, influential and supportive, and I have learnt so much from them.

I am a big movie fan, so actors and movie characters, like Sylvester Stallone in *Rocky*, Arnold Schwarzenegger in *Predator*, Robin Williams in *Mrs Doubtfire*, Bruce Lee in *Enter The Dragon*, all inspire me, for their struggles against adversity, both on and off the screen. For their courage, to put themselves out there, to be vulnerable, and to never give up. I am also a massive sports fan. Icons like Roger Federer, Rafael Nadal, Novak Djokovic, Billie Jean King, Martina Navratilova, Jana Novotna, Lewis Hamilton, and Michael Jordan. Their amazing ability to adapt and be resilient, and to keep on improving, meant that they all motivated and inspired me. When things get tough for me, I ask myself, what would these guys do in this situation? This really helps ignite that spark to keep moving forwards.

Before the operation, I chose to be the hero of my story, focusing on famous people that resonated with me. Tap into all the heroes you look up to, and ask what they would do during tough times. Who are your heroes? Create your own story and keep pushing forward.

I was now in good place, ready as much as I could be, for the operation.

CHAPTER 6
THE DAY OF SURGERY

It was Friday, September 30th 2016. The day of the operation had finally arrived. My alarm went off at 5.15am, and I slowly awoke from a restless sleep. I had a whole mixture of thoughts and feelings, from excitement that I could finally get the cancer removed, to fearful anticipation of what was to come.

I felt strong, focused and calm as I looked in the mirror. Whilst brushing my teeth I repeated internally to myself, "I CAN do this, I can DO this, I can do THIS".

After an amazing long shower, I double checked the contents of my small and medium-sized sports bags, before going downstairs to say good morning to mum, dad and my two younger brothers.

I only had a glass of water as I had to remain nil by mouth. This was all I was allowed to have prior to the operation.

The weather was dull and grey, but the air smelt fresh as we made our way to the hospital. It was a quiet drive of about 30 minutes. The family were all in their own thoughts, managing and coping the best that they could. On the way to the hospital, I was thinking to myself, how grateful I was to have the NHS and my family there, fully supporting me to overcome this challenge. I also felt proud of myself, because I had prepared myself mentally and emotionally to be positive, and believed that everything would work out. I had visualised a successful surgery, and had taken steps to set myself up to succeed.

ARRIVING AT THE HOSPITAL

We arrived at Northwick Hospital, Admissions Ward, at 7am. We were early and the reception had not yet opened. We waited with other patients in the reception area. I assumed that some of them would also be having an operation today. Once the reception opened at 7.30am, I checked in. My family and I were then guided to the admissions ward and I was allocated a hospital bed.

MEETING THE MEDICAL TEAM AND FINAL OP PREP

I met my doctor and the medical team. I was happy, smiley, cheerful and really grateful that they were here to help me. I have to say that they were also happy too, which was really nice to see, and made me feel at ease. The doctor analysed my mouth to see how things were. He was surprised by how big the tumour had grown, since he'd last seen me, and expressed that everything would be okay.

I did have some internal nerves, but I immediately put these in check, by acknowledging that this was the best course of action. I told myself to stay focused on each of the steps that were to follow. This is how I kept calm and present, without any overthinking.

I got dressed into the hospital gown and also put on some surgical stockings, which are designed to prevent any blood clots.

The medical team then proceeded with the following pre-operation checks:

• Taking my blood pressure.

• Checking the details were correct for the identification wrist bands, with my full name and date of birth, and then placing them on my non-operating limbs.

• Marking the donor arm so that the skin could be taken to form the flap. I am right arm dominant, and so chose to have my left arm as the donor arm. (Some patients have the skin taken from the lower leg, dependent on what the doctors will advise).

• Marking which nostril I wanted the nasogastric tube (NG) to be in. I chose my left nostril, as I felt that I breathe more easily through my right nostril.

We were now ready to go for the operation. I hugged my mum, dad and brothers and we exchanged positive words, and I said that I would see them tomorrow. I gave the nurse my small bag to look after, and took the small Zohar book with me. I was given a choice to walk or wheeled on the bed to the operating theatre – I chose to walk.

I was led into a room where the anaesthetic team transferred me to another bed. The bed had a lovely warm inflatable mattress, and I was then covered with a warm foiled blanket. I felt really warm and cosy. Whilst the team were getting me ready to have the general anaesthetic, I had a nice chat with one of the doctors about hobbies. I talked about tennis and how I had played the game for over 30 years. I felt calm and relaxed, in positive spirits. I gave the doctor my small book and she said that she would place it near my bed during the operation. The doctor then advised that they would start to proceed with giving me the anaesthetic, and then I would slowly fall asleep.

Once in a deep sleep, I was then taken to the operating theatre, where the operation would take approximately 12 hours.

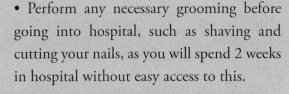

• Perform any necessary grooming before going into hospital, such as shaving and cutting your nails, as you will spend 2 weeks in hospital without easy access to this.

• Focus on your positive affirmations and visualisations. Remember this operation is going to help you.

• Don't forget to take your smaller bag

• I also recommend that the medical team

have your parents/loved ones' phone contact details, so that they can call them once the operation is finished.

 • Also, I advise that your parents/loved ones, should have the hospital and medical team's phone numbers, so that they can call, just in case they are not notified when the operation is finished.

Letting go and having complete faith and trust in the medical team, also helped me during this time. I believed in the process and knew that I'd prepared myself as much as I could, for success. I would not know the outcome of the operation until I woke up and heard from the medical team. That would be my next step, and I would do my best to be ready for that moment.

CHAPTER 7
POST OPERATION,
INTENSIVE CARE UNIT

I was slowly and gently woken up from the anaesthetic, by one of the doctors. As my eyes opened it was very bright, I felt slightly groggy, as if I was waking up from a nice long sleep, and I did not know where I was. The nurse then said that I was in the Intensive Care Unit (ICU).

I thought to myself, have I had the operation yet, or are we about to go and have the operation? The nurse informed me that I had indeed had the operation and that it had gone well. I mumbled okay and said thanks. I could actually speak a little, which was great. I took a deep breath in, looked up to the sky, (well, the ceiling,) and said Thank You, and then breathed out with a peaceful sigh. I was simultaneously relieved and grateful, that the surgery had been completed. My next words, to the nurse, were, "I need to meditate and could I have some shades for my eyes as the lights are very, very bright." I did not know why I said this. I think I had conditioned myself over the past few weeks to remain calm and meditation was the key. The doctor improvised and provided some protective glasses with pieces of paper over the lenses, and placed them over my eyes. I then shut my eyes and rested.

 You can use the eye mask that I recommended in an earlier chapter, which you added to your small bag.

THE ICU

The ICU is for the patients who have recently had an operation, and are placed under intensive care and close supervision. The environment is very clean and clinical and somewhat quiet. I was introduced to some of the nurses on shift who would look after me. They informed me that I had two buttons which I could press. One was for alerting the nurse and the other was for dispensing morphine for pain. The latter only worked every 5 minutes. My state of mind at the time was that I did not want to experience any pain and was not going to wait for it to happen, so I proceeded to press the button every 5 minutes. In retrospect, this might not have been a good idea, as you will see.

MY APPEARANCE

I was lying on my back with pillows propped up behind me, in a bed at a 35% incline, with my left arm heavily bandaged and elevated at my side on top of a pillow. I had tubes coming out of nose, neck, chest, stomach, penis and left lower arm. My neck was heavily patched as well the left side of my stomach.

Please see illustration below:

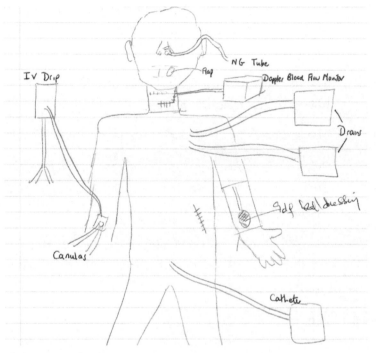

Whilst this may look worrying, I was not fully aware of how I looked at the time.

- The NG Tube, in my nose(down my oesophagus and into my stomach), was there to feed me.

- The see-through neck patching was there to protect and heal the neck after being dissected and then stitched together.

- The wire protruding from my neck and connecting to the Doppler Blood Flow monitor was there to check that there was blood flow to the flap, via the vein which was removed from my left arm.

- The drains were there to capture any remaining blood or fluids near the operated parts, of the neck and drain them safely.

- The intravenous drip was there to hydrate, provide nutrition and monitor volumes of fluid input.

- The catheter was there to allow urine to pass and to also monitor the volumes of fluid output.

- The canula was there so that medication could be given or bloods could be taken.

Over the course of my stay in hospital I realized that all of the above were there to help me recover and get better. I accepted this and tried my best to get comfortable.

HOW I FELT

There were a number of challenges that made me feel unsettled:

- I was very uncomfortable having to remain on my back at a 35 degrees incline. I could not turn my head left or right, as my neck was heavily dressed. I also could not turn on my side, as I normally do, when I lie down. This added to my discomfort and was why I could not sleep.

- The left hand side of my mouth was quite sore, this was where the doctors had to stretch and open my mouth wide to operate on my tongue.

  Recommendation: Use Lip Balm, which was added to the small bag, or alternatively you can use the Lanolin that the nurses provide. Personally, I found the lip balm was better.

- Back to the morphine – After having a number of doses of morphine I was unsure whether or not it helped. What I can say is that as soon as I moved my body one way, my stomach liquids moved, and then all of a sudden I vomited. This was a side effect of having too much morphine. From that point onwards, I stopped taking the morphine.

- Whenever I tried shutting my eyes, my mind played out these fast cartoon animations – they were really fast flickering pictures – but I couldn't work out the characters. It was as if my mind was in overdrive. This could have been the side effects of the anaesthetic and morphine, which also inhibited my sleep.

- I was coughing up a lot of secretions throughout the day and night. This was continuous. I was given a suction tube to help suck away the secretions. I had to use this a lot and endure through it, knowing that it would get better after 7 to 9 days. I had to take it one day at a time, and think, if I can get through this day, then it's one step closer to recovery.

- Overall, I felt quite restless, as I could not get comfortable nor sleep. It was very challenging dealing with this discomfort.

- The positive news was that my mouth and tongue, were not causing me any pain.

HOW I OVERCAME THE DISCOMFORT

Here are a few observations of my attempts to overcome the discomfort:

- There were no real solutions. I had to accept the situation and think to myself - things will get better. I just tried to rest when I could.

- Once I was in the ICU I was fully reliant on the nurses looking after me. They did an amazing job taking care of me. I had to accept that I was no longer in control and placed my trust in the nurses. This was a new experience for me and I had no choice but to accept it and go with it.

- In retrospect, I think perhaps having some music to listen to may have helped me to relax and pass the time more easily. I did receive my small bag from the nurse, which had my mobile phone, but I did not use it as I was quite restless and found it difficult to focus.

- The nurses provided Paracetamol for pain management. They also provided a Nebuilser, which helped to bring up all the secretions. Both of these did help to ease the discomfort.

FAMILY VISIT

My family did visit me late on Friday night, after the operation. However, I do not remember this, and I put this down to the anaesthetic.

Whilst in ICU I witnessed other families having loved ones going through trauma. But I knew it was important to manage my emotions and stay concentrated on my own recovery.

PROGRESS UPDATE BY DOCTORS

On Saturday, early in the afternoon, the doctors came to see how I was doing. They said that the operation had gone really well. They advised me that during the operation they'd found the cancer to be a lot deeper than expected and also found that the cancer was located at the base of my tongue, which was not visible on the scans. Based on these findings, they increased the staging of the cancer from 2 to 4. They also expressed that they had successfully removed all of the cancer, which was excellent news. The neck dissection and the removal of 57 lymph nodes was also successful and the results of the histology would take one week.

A week later, I got the histology results, and it was very good news. They hadn't found any cancer in my lymph nodes, which meant that it had not spread to other parts of my body, and was only local. I was so happy and relieved, and shouted 'yes', internally. I also said thank you, to that someone, up in the sky.

OBSERVATION

If the MRI and CT Scanning technology was improved, with better magnification and detection of cancerous cells, they would have been able to determine if the lymph nodes had cancer or not, and thus I would have avoided unnecessary surgery, because neck dissection may not have been required, which would have avoided any post-surgery side effects. One doctor expressed that scanning technology can only detect cancer when there are at least 100,000 cancer cells. That's a lot of cells, so there is definitely room for improvement here, to improve the quality of scanning technology and thus the quality of life for patients. I am confident that this will improve in the near future.

WALKING

On Saturday morning, around 9.30am, I phoned home to check what time my parents and brothers would visit. I was keen to see them so that they could brighten up my day, after another sleepless night.

Soon after, one of the male nurses was there to help me get out of bed and start slowly walking. All of the tubes had to be carefully organized so that they did not get tangled, when I got out of bed. There were a number of progressive steps to do this, all assisted, and these were as follows:

- The first step was to move from the bed and sit upright in a chair. This took a while to get used to as I had been lying down for such a long time. The nurse clamped the drains to my gown, and put my slippers on, which came from my small bag.

- The second step was to get me standing on my feet. The nurse made sure I was balanced and feeling okay.

- Then the third, was to slowly walk, with the nurse standing by.

Walking slowly towards the other end of the ward, I realized that there were large windows looking out to trees and daylight. Seeing the outside and nature made me feel absolutely amazing. My whole mood picked up. Walking slowly, up and down the ward, felt great. Yes, I may have been a little weak, but I felt like I was making some good progress and it was great to be out of bed.

The male nurse that helped me was amazing at putting me at ease and was very patient and caring. I am very grateful for his help.

TOUGH NIGHT

I found it very tough, in the early hours of Sunday morning. It was another night without sleep, I was feeling mentally fatigued and was continuously coughing up secretions. Having to use the suction every few minutes, broke up any sleep. Especially as I had to be focused, making sure I was very careful, only using the suction on the side of the mouth that was not operated on. I felt very helpless and restless. I felt powerless because I could do absolutely nothing about the constant secretions. I almost broke down in tears, but I managed to hold it together.

There was a part of me that felt very isolated and alone. I knew it was all on me to overcome this. I thought to myself that it would not help if I broke down in that moment, so I chose to shut my eyes and breathe slowly through my nose. I focused on relaxing and being more patient. I tried to slow everything down, build more calmness within and have a positive outward focus, in the next steps of my recovery. I knew that releasing emotion could indeed be quite freeing, but I was just not willing to do this. I think this is a personal choice, and you have to go with what works for you in the moment you are in. I also realized that what I was thinking and feeling could be all part of the effects that both morphine and the anaesthetic have, and I tried to be kinder to myself.

CATHETER EPISODE

On Sunday, the nurse was concerned that the fluid volumes going into my body did not match the volume output from the catheter bag. They decided that they had to remove the tube from my penis and replace it with a new one. Being awake for this was not an ideal experience, but I have to say it was not that bad. So if you have to go through this, know that it will be okay. The irony was that on Monday they actually decided to remove the catheter permanently. I saw the funny side to this and just had to smile about the whole thing.

TWO DAYS AFTER THE OPERATION

On Sunday morning I continued to get up and sit in the chair and also walk up and down the ward, assisted by the nurse. I was feeling stronger and better within myself.

Late on Sunday afternoon, the doctors said I was now ready to be moved to the general ward. This was fantastic news. It was progress and my spirits rose.

The ICU Ward can feel very isolated and clinical. My recommendation is, if you can move to the General Ward sooner, then do so. Of course, this is based on the doctor's recommendation. As soon as I reached the General Ward, I felt so much better as I met other patients who'd had similar operations and there were just more people around. It made me feel emotionally and mentally better and more connected.

CHAPTER 8
RECOVERY IN THE
GENERAL WARD

Being transferred to the General Ward really helped to boost my spirits. It was great to be amongst more people. The Gray Ward, at Northwick Park Hospital, "treats diseases that affect the face, jaw, mouth, teeth, neck, salivary glands and skin. This includes treating deformities of the face, facial injuries and serious infections of the head and neck."

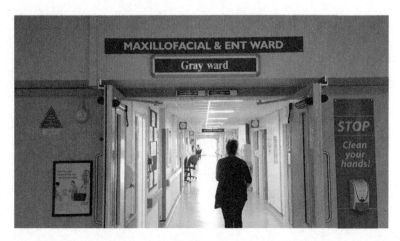

This would be my home for the next 11.5 days, before being discharged from hospital.

I was assigned to a 4-bed ward, bay A3, in the right-hand corner of the room, next to the window. Outside, there was a lovely view of Wembley Stadium.

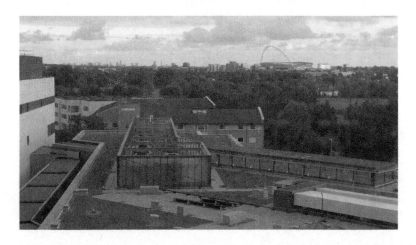

Having a beautiful view of the trees and greenery made me realise what a wonderful world there was out there, and that I still had a lot of great living to do. This kept me positive and focused on getting better.

In the ward there were two other patients. One gentleman had a tracheostomy and the other had a similar operation to me, except the skin flap for the tongue reconstruction had been taken from his left calf rather than the arm. I smiled and nodded at both of them, and they did the same. It was an acknowledgement of respect and understanding, that we were all going through the same thing.

During my stay, there were many activities that were all part of my recovery process, which I will discuss next. I have also expressed what I felt, along with what practical and positive actions I took to improve things for myself. I hope you find them useful.

PERSONAL LOCKERS

The bay on the General Ward had a personal locker, for me to put my belongings in. My parents brought my medium-sized bag to the hospital on the Monday, so I was able to put some of the essential daily items that I would use into the locker. These included my journal and pens, reading books, mobile phone and charger, headphones, ear plugs and toiletry bag. Below, you can see the locker space, as well a lot of electrical power points behind the bed.

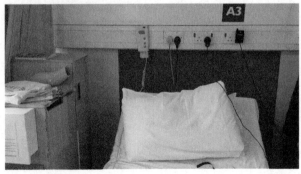

FROTH OF THE DOG

During the 10 to 12 hour surgery, my salivary excretions were somehow stored or inhibited. The side effect of this was that once the operation was done, I found that I was bringing up all of these excretions. Throughout my first night in the general ward, I was bringing up a lot of salivary excretions and was constantly seeking assistance from the nurses to adjust the incline of the bed so that I could cope better, as well as seeking help in using the suction tube.

After the operation (Day 1) through to Day 8 of recovery, I found that I could not stop bringing up saliva. I kept 'frothing' at the mouth, like Cujo the dog, from the Stephen King movie. Despite trying to stay positive at this time, I did find this unbearable.

The best advice I can give, is that it is better out than in. I was supplied with a suction tube, lots of tissues and many cardboard containers to use, so that I could suction up or cough up the salivary excretions.

There were many times I felt very helpless, as I had no control over this. Another major difficulty was that I couldn't sleep because I was constantly suctioning up or coughing up saliva. Swallowing is another option, but I needed to get the excess saliva out of my body.

I was provided with a face mask to breathe into, called a "nebuliser". It contained sodium chloride, which helped to loosen up all the secretions and therefore get them out. I kept using this, and it helped a great deal.

Sometimes, during family visits, I wanted to talk, but every time I tried, the secretions just kept coming out of my mouth. There was absolutely nothing I could do, but to accept it and know that it would get better. I would take in deep breaths, and a focus on a positive future. I kept telling myself, "I can do this, it is getting better", which really helped me through it.

The secretions will stop eventually. It took up to 8 or 9 days, so if you experience the same thing, keep positive and know that it will go.

DROOLING

After the operation, it is normal for the tongue and mouth to be swollen and numb. I had this and found it hard to close my mouth fully. I noticed that when I dropped off to sleep and then woke up, that I had saliva dripping down my mouth and neck, onto the gown. Yes, it was annoying and unsightly, but again I accepted this, as I knew this would be temporary. I made an adjustment and placed tissues under my chin, and then later on, I used a flannel to capture the drool.

MONITORING BLOOD FLOW TO THE FLAP

The vein, taken from my arm, was connected to the blood supply in my neck, and to the flap that had been stitched to my tongue. The flap consists of living and breathing tissue, and needs a blood supply to stay healthy. During the next 9 days, post-operation, the doctors monitored the blood flow to the flap, using a Doppler Blood Flow Monitor Machine.

They also asked me to monitor the flap throughout the day. This was very important. The flap is at high risk, post-op. Over a period of 5 days, it could lose blood supply and die, which would mean that another reconstructive surgery to fix

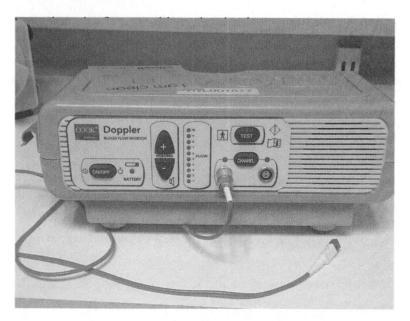

I was very focused, cautious and somewhat paranoid about this risk, and made sure that I regularly checked the blood flow to my flap. This was achieved by turning on the Doppler Machine and connecting the protruding silver wire from my neck, which extended to a long reel of blue coloured covered wire (see below), to the machine. A sound would be heard if there was blood flow to the flap.

 I recommend checking the blood flow regularly, at least for your peace of mind.

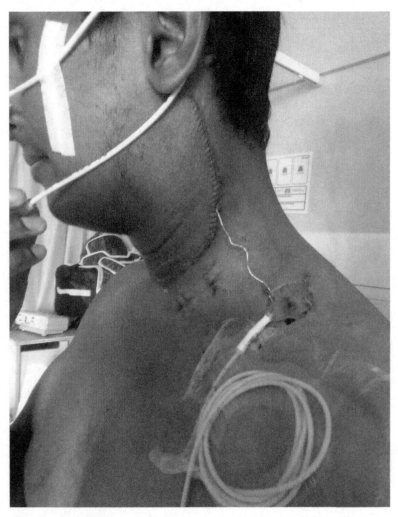

DAY 4 PROGRESS

On my first morning in the general ward, I woke up to a brand new day and I felt good. Looking out of the window, it was bright with blue skies and very peaceful. The nurses assisted me with a sponge bath and changed my gown and stockings for fresh ones. This was the first time since surgery that I was having a wash. I had gotten used to the smell of dried blood, but it was great to have that washed away. I felt much better for being cleaner and fresher.

The doctors came round for their morning checkups and they were very happy with my progress. They advised the nurses to remove the drain from my leg, the intravenous drip and also the catheter. This was fantastic. I saw this as wonderful progress and wrote in my journal about the wonderful positive news. This made me feel very happy.

DAILY ROUTINES

I like daily routines, as they give me structure and purpose to the day. In the table below, I have listed out some of the key activities that happened during the day in the General Ward.

8am/8.15am - Nurses received handover of patients from nightshift.

8.30am/9.15am - Doctors walked round to see each patient – a great opportunity to write any questions down to ask them beforehand.

8.45am/9.30am - Nurse gave medications.

9.am - Sat in the chair whilst the nurse changed the bed, provided a towel and a new gown and sometimes new compression stockings, to prevent DVT.

10am -1pm - Nurse helped with bathing, or a shower if capable.

10am – 1pm - Nebuliser provided.

10am -1pm - Start food feed via NG tube.

1.15pm - Nurse gave 3 water flushes through NG tube.

4.45pm - Nurse took blood pressure and body temperature.

6pm - Nurse gave medications.

9.15pm - Nurse gave medications.

9.20pm - Nebuliser provided.

9.30pm - Nurse took blood pressure and body temperature.

9.40pm - Handover to nightshift nurses, and also doctors on nightshift performed check-ups. They checked mouth/flap and blood flow to flap via Doppler machine.

In between all of these activities, I was either resting, sleeping or walking up and down the ward.

DAILY MEDICATIONS

The medications that I was on are detailed below. These were prescribed by doctors and provided by the nurses. I did find that, after a while, they made me constipated – so having the lactulose helped to improve this.

Morning

- 2 Paracetamol

- 1 Ibuprofen (optional)

- 1 Lactulose (optional)

- 1 Nebuliser

- 4 Water flushes 60 ml each

Evening

- 2 Paracetamol

- 1 Ibuprofen or Codeine (optional) – I was given codeine when I had more pain of discomfort in swallowing

- 1 Lactulose (optional)

- 1 Nebuliser

- 1 Blood Thinner Injection

GOING TO THE TOILET BY MYSELF

With the catheter out on day 4, I was now able to go to the toilet by myself. That first time that I went, after the op, I was getting used to using my muscles again. It was an effort and there was a burning sensation as well. Nevertheless, I was doing this by myself and it felt like good progress.

On my first trip to the toilet, this was the first time that I could wash my hands. The feeling of water running on my hands was wonderful. Just being able to walk to the bathroom and run cold water over my hands made me feel so amazing, and I was really appreciating the small things in life.

It was also the first time that I could look in a big mirror and see my face. I saw how swollen the left-hand side of my face, jaw and neck were. I also opened my mouth to see what it looked like. I was absolutely amazed at seeing the flap and tongue for the first time. It was a 'wow' moment. I do not know how the doctors do this, but they are really something special. I was very happy with how it looked. Yes, it was swollen, but I knew that this would eventually reduce and go down.

Looking in the mirror, I also looked into my own eyes. I mean really looked into my eyes to see what was there. I saw me. Yes, I was still there. I saw kindness, gratitude, and appreciation for still being me. I also saw a strength of steel and resilience, knowing that I had a wonderful opportunity to recover and make my life into a spectacular one, even more so than before. Again, I was chanting to myself, "Yes, I can do this."

It was an amazing feeling to be able to go to the toilet by myself. This was something that I could control, and it made me feel like I was recovering well and starting to live more, by doings things for myself. I would take every small bit of progress and I would write about this improvement in my journal.

SMELLY MOUTH

It was Day 5 and my mouth had not yet been cleaned since the surgery. I had not drunk anything as I was still on IV Fluids.

This was because the doctors wanted to allow enough time for the tongue to heal. However, my mouth was very smelly, with yellow gunge on the side of the mouth that was operated on. In fact, my mum could smell it from 5 metres away. The doctors advised that I could clean this very delicately, using small rectangular "pink sponge" soft brushes. They look like a small lollipop stick and are prescribed to you by the hospital. I actually found these too large to use, so I cut sponges in half. My mum helped to clean my mouth delicately, as I could not see what I was doing. Sometimes the mouth would bleed as the sponge brushed over some stitching, so we had to be very careful.

In the following days I was allowed to dip the pink sponge brushes in some Corsodyl mouthwash and clean the mouth lightly. I was able to do this by myself, as I had a small torch and a mirror, so that I could see what I was doing.

DAYS 5 AND 6

There was lots of progress over these two days. I had two drains removed from my chest. I also had an X-ray of my chest, to make sure there was no fluid in one of my lungs. I'm happy to say that there was no fluid. I also was moved to a 6 bed ward, Bay C2, within Gray Ward, for less intensive care patients.

You can see from the picture opposite that I had my bag on top of the locker for easier access, and also a side table next to my bed with medications, containers and tissues at hand. On my bed, if you look closely, I have my black journal and a newspaper.

Moving to another room felt like I was again making small steps of progress. In this bay there were 6 other patients, including myself. Being in fresh surroundings, bred a fresh perspective. I was feeling stronger and more alive.

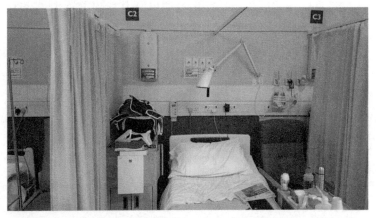

I also started walking a lot more, up and down the main hallway of Gray Ward. I had more freedom of movement, without the drains. At one end of the hallway there was a window, slightly open, with a view of the car park and landscape. Breathing in the fresh air and scenery was a great feeling. I had a feeling of gratitude and happiness that I was getting better.

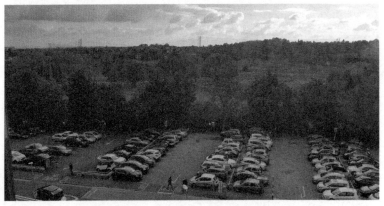

DIETICIANS AND NUTRITION

Immediately after having the operation my mouth needed to heal. I was fed through a tube that was inserted through my left nostril, down the oesophagus into the stomach (called a Nasogastric (NG) Tube) for the next 12 days. The dieticians prescribed a 2000 calorie milk shake called TwoCal. This drink would provide all the nutrients I needed to sustain myself and build me up. I would be given the TwoCal shake once a day, and it would take 3 to 4 hours to drip feed me. Sometimes during the feed, I would feel some of the shake come up into my throat, which was not a nice feeling, and made me feel nauseous. I soon realised that lying at 30 degrees on the bed while feeding may not have helped. I should have sat upright in a chair, or stood up, during the feed – so that gravity could help the shake to pass down easily into the stomach. I did not digest the TwoCal shake very well, so the dieticians changed the milkshake to one that was less thick and slightly less calorific, which was much better. Additionally, between the feed, I would have water flushes to help wash down the shake. When I was in discomfort, I would have a water flush.

SPEECH AND LANGUAGE THERAPISTS (SALT)

The SALT team also checked in on me to see how I was doing. They looked at the movement of my mouth and tongue and also listened to my speech. They said I was sounding pretty good, and that they could understand me. That was great, because deep down inside I did think about whether I would be able to fully speak again. They also checked on my swallowing action. This was important, because the swallowing muscles can weaken quite quickly if not used regularly. This can happen post-op, as I was using the NG tube instead of swallowing.

NG TUBE DISCOMFORT

Whilst the NG tube was there to feed me, I could not really get used to it. I did find it quite uncomfortable and found that it generated a tickly cough from time to time. The worst part about it was that I found it painful to swallow sometimes. It's like my body knew that the NG tube should not really be there, and that it was obstructing part of my oesophagus, but I knew I just had to adapt somehow. I found that if I tilted my neck slightly forward this helped to reduce the discomfort in swallowing.

If there is discomfort swallowing with an NG tube in place, I recommend varying the neck angle to find a position where swallowing is easier. I just told myself that the NG tube would be removed in 10 to 13 days' time, and that it was temporary, so I could accept it and take it one day at a time.

WATER FLUSHES

One of the best parts of my day was when the nurse flushed 4x 60ml syringes of water through the NG tube, into my stomach. There was a cooling and soothing sensation, of the water going down my throat and into my stomach. This gave me some sense of relief and made things feel less uncomfortable. I highly recommend having this when you are finding it difficult to cope and want a pick-me-up.

SLEEP

The following impeded my sleep:

• I had lots of neck dressings on the front of my neck, which made my neck very stiff and uncomfortable.

• I also had my left arm bandage from where the skin and vein for the flap was taken.

• The NG tube made it a little painful to swallow, as mentioned above.

• Lying on my back at a 40 degree elevation was very uncomfortable for my back and shoulders. The lack of movement did not help.

• The nurses took my blood pressure and body temperature every 4 hours.

IMPROVEMENTS ON SLEEP

• I would get 3-4 water flushes at night. Sometimes I just could not sleep, as I was in discomfort for the above reasons. I found that the water flushes helped me to drop off. I had to go to the toilet a couple of times at night, either using a urinal or going to the bathroom, but it was worth it.

• On Day 10, the doctor removed the neck dressing. This had severely restricted my movement to either side, whilst the stitching in my neck was healing. Once removed I felt so much better and could sleep a lot easier.

• Removal of all drains provided more freedom of movement whilst sleeping. With both the neck patching and drains removed, I could sleep on my side like I normally do.

• Visualising all the future activities I wanted to do and also chanting my affirmations in my head, made things a lot better as well.

• Focusing on one day at a time, and not overthinking about what was to come, really helped the days to go quicker. For example, I just kept thinking that if I can get through this day, then it's one step closer to recovery.

ACTIVITIES

READING, MUSIC AND MOVIES

I had a few books and magazines to read during my two-week stay in hospital. I was reading *Healing and Recovery* by David R. Hawkins, to help me understand how I can help myself to get better. I was also reading *The Secret* by Rhonda Byrne. Both these books stimulated my mind.

Listening to music helped to relax and calm me, and was also a great way to get me to sleep. I also listened to body scan meditations, which kept me in touch with my breathing and awareness of how I felt.

The Gray Ward has a small TV room, which I would use from time to time. This would help break up the monotony of being in bed or within the ward. Other times, I would try to watch a movie on my mobile phone. I made a choice not to use any social media, as I felt this would not serve me and would be more of a negative distraction.

JOURNALING

Journaling played a big part in helping me to cope, and I would write in my journal every day. I would write about the thoughts I was having, documenting every bit of progress I was making, from drains being removed to my strength and energy improving. I also noted down my questions each day, prior to doctor's morning and evening rounds, in readiness for them to answer.

These included questions and requests such as:

• Are the stitches on my tongue dissolvable? Or do they need to be removed?

• Can I start to brush my teeth lightly with toothpaste?

• When do you think the swelling of the tongue will go down?

• Can you confirm if the mouth has fully healed?

• Can you check if my flap is okay?

• I sometimes cough up the TwoCal milkshake, is this acid reflux?

• Is the Doppler sound okay?

• Please can you secure my NG line on my nose?

• I have not opened my bowels for 3 days, please could you advise?

• I'm still bringing up secretions, when will this stop?

• Can you ask the doctor if it is okay to gargle with diluted Corsodyl?

• I need help cleaning my mouth.

I wrote down every bit of progress that was being made. This helped me tremendously, and it made me feel like I was improving.

DAYDREAMING

There were times where I spent a lot of time day dreaming and zoning out, thinking about if it was all worth it. I think this was because I had hardly got any sleep due to being in one form of discomfort or another. However, I would always refer back to my visions for the future, my affirmations and also realising that this operation was the only choice I had to heal from the cancer. I think bouncing from accepting and making peace with my situation, to asking why me and worrying about things is completely natural. Eventually, I would get back to focusing on my visions for the future and affirmations, knowing that things would get better.

NIGHT TIME

Lying in bed, there were times when I felt like I was going to break down with emotion, because sometimes it was just too tough and overwhelming. But I knew that this would not serve me. I had to remain strong, not only for me, but for my family. I would eventually have an emotional release, later in my recovery, which I will express later in the book (see Chapter 12 - UPW Crewing).

Sometimes at night, other patients would go through a tough time and were quite vocal. In order for me to focus on my health and sleep, I used ear plugs and an eye mask to block out the sound and light, which helped me improve my sleep and cope better.

DESTRUCTIVE TIMES

There was one instance during the night when I was moving in and out of sleep. I was quite restless and frustrated. I felt that enough was enough and I just wanted to go home. I realized and accepted that it was okay to feel this way. My mindset was negative at the time, but then the thought hit me – this is not going to help me. I decided right then and there to journal my thoughts. I got out my journal and started writing. I find that getting my thoughts on a page helps to channel the frustration and the irritability, via movement and activity. It helps me to change the state I am in. I then changed my focus, and wrote who I was and what I looked forward to.

 Write down who you are and why you want to live. Get clarity on this, and it will help you regain your strength and focus for your recovery. It will also help you in the inevitable dark moments.

In that moment, I started to feel much better. I took a few deep breaths and I thought about this second opportunity I had been given to live a great life, spend more time with family and friends, help and serve others, and travel to lots of wonderful new places. A second opportunity to do the things I loved to do. I was back to my positive self and went back to sleep. Again, I think you go with what works for you. It is okay to emotionally release and vent, and then eventually get to a point where you have accepted the situation and then reset, in a more peaceful state.

DAILY VISITS AND MASSAGES

I would look forward to my parents and immediate family coming to visit me. Sometimes they would come in the early afternoon and then again in the evening. It was great to have this amazing support, and it was such an important part of my recovery. I am so grateful to them, it really meant a lot.

Because I spent a lot of time lying down, and was not using my shoulder or back muscles, I had a build up of a lot of knots and tension. I found this very uncomfortable. My mum was a life saver, as she would give me a back and shoulder massage every day, using aromatherapy oils. This made such a big difference. I found that I could rest and sleep much better later that day.

I also brought with me a small massage ball. I placed this between a wall and my back and shoulders and rolled it slowly over areas that were tight and knotted. I did this throughout the day to help loosen those areas and make me feel more relaxed.

I recommend getting a daily back massage from family or friends. I think this is so important in the recovery process, and if family members can't do it, then I would ask if you can get support from the hospital to do this.

VIDEO MESSAGES FROM FRIENDS

My brother came up with an excellent idea whilst I was in the general ward. He would send me a video message every day, via WhatsApp, from friends, wishing me a speedy recovery and lots of love and support.

This was very powerful and kept my spirits up and moving forwards. It helped me to realise that I had so much to live for, and so many friends to catch up with after I had recovered.

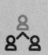

When friends ask how they can help you I recommend that you ask them to send you a short video message. It will boost your spirits!

GET WELL CARDS

I received a lot of cards from family and friends. This was great. Some of the cards were very humorous and made me laugh. They made me feel really good inside, and made me feel mentally stronger, so I could get better, and meet up with all of them very soon.

PHYSIO

On Day 8, the physio came to meet me, to discuss exercises that would help restore mobility and strength in my left shoulder, arm, hand and neck. I found that all of these areas were very stiff, tight and somewhat sore. Here are some of the things I experienced:

• I could not snap my fingers, thumb and middle finger, in my left hand, like I used to.

• The mobility of my thumb was weak.

• I could not straighten my left arm out to the side, as my left-hand side of my neck and shoulder was weak and very tight. In fact, my left arm would shake and quiver with effort when I tried to do this.

• I found it difficult to rotate my left arm, from my palm facing the ground to turning it around, to facing the ceiling, and then vice versa.

This was a lot to take in, as I was thinking about how this could impact me when playing tennis. Playing tennis is one of my passions and I have a two handed backhand, which requires a lot of strength and movement with the left arm. I switched my thoughts around and told myself that at least I have some movement, and so it would eventually get better. I just had to keep exercising it and take it one day at a time.

Here are some of the exercises that were recommended:

SHOULDERS

• Squeeze the shoulder blades down and back together.

• Hold for 10 seconds.

• Repeat 10 times (as pain allows).

NECK

My neck was extremely tight after surgery. The stitching was beautifully done as shown in the photo opposite.

I was encouraged to perform the following neck exercises to get move movement in that area:

• Tuck chin to chest.

• Look up to the ceiling.

• Turn head to look over right shoulder.

• Turn head to look over left shoulder.

• Increase turn as pain allows.

• Tilt head to bring right ear to right shoulder.

• Tilt head to bring left ear to left shoulder.

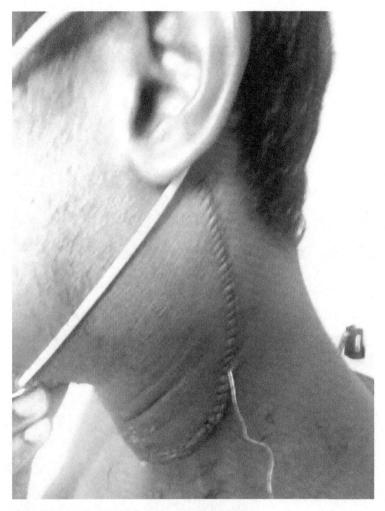

EXERCISE LEFT ARM, BACK & SHOULDERS

With the lack of use of my left side, my upper back and shoulders developed muscle atrophy. This happened whilst I was recovering both inside and out of the hospital, and happened up to 6 weeks after surgery.

Here are some pictures:

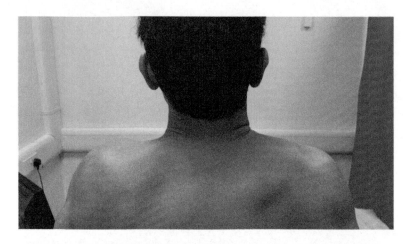

From this picture you can see the dip on my left shoulder, where the muscle on my left trap has withered away, in comparison to my right trap. It's true, if you do not use it, you lose it. You can also see that the middle back muscles are not there.

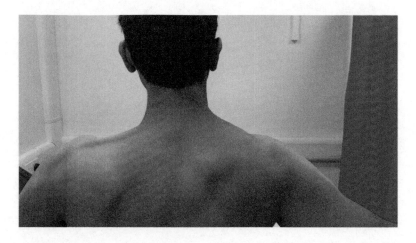

In this picture I have slightly straightened out my arms laterally.

You can actually see the small line of muscle on top of my left shoulder, and again the lack of muscle on my left middle back.

I am not sure what the doctors can do here to help patients to reduce muscle atrophy whilst we are in recovery. It might be that we have to wait for our mouth, arm and neck to heal before they recommend any specific exercises to address the atrophy.

I would recommend, and please check with your doctor, to try and do some left shoulder and back exercises, just to use those muscles. Doing some light seated pulls, just to keep the muscles awake, might go a long way. The sooner you can do some of these exercises, the less likely you are to develop muscle atrophy.

LEFT ARM

Hand: Move all fingers.

Make a fist and then open and close.

Wrist: Move up and down.

Arm: Turn arm over so that palm faces up and then down.

I also continued to use my massage ball to massage my upper back and shoulders against the wall.

DAY 8 - GOLF BALL DRESSING

On Day 8, as well as seeing the physio, I had the dressing removed from my tummy and also the bandage from my left arm. The tummy had healed well. This is where they took part of the skin from my tummy, stitched this up, and then stitched this section of skin over the skin that was removed from my left hand, for the flap. Again, this was amazing from the surgeons.

I called it a "golf ball" dressing. It is actually a sponged dressing that is stapled to my skin. You can see the staples on the circumference of the dressing. Above the dressing you can also see the long line of scarring, where the vein was taken and placed in my neck, sending blood to the flap.

This is what my arm looked like:

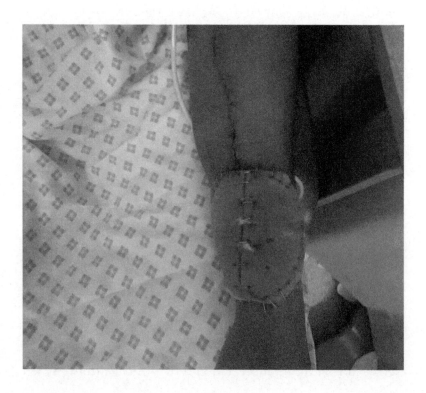

As I am talking about the golf ball, let me skip to Day 10, when they removed this dressing. The nurse had to use scissors to cut the staples off. This was a little painful and I just had to suck it up. I tried to look at the funny side of this – like, is this really happening? I smiled and laughed as the nurse cut the staples. This was the easy part. The next step was for the nurse to tweeze the staple out of my skin in the arm, carefully. This was not so bad, as I think my arm was numbed before we did this. Once the staples were removed, the sponge dressing was removed. As the nurse removed it, I could see all the moisture and fluids that had been absorbed by the sponge. My arm was then revealed, and this is what I saw:

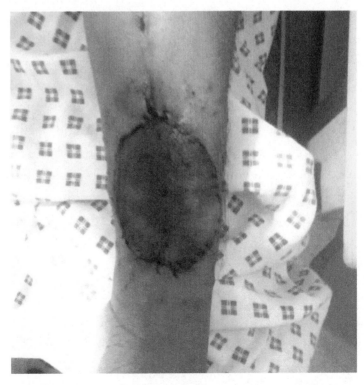

This oval shaped, very bruised looking, section of skin, had come from my tummy and had been proficiently and delicately stitched to my arm – unbelievable. I'll say it again, surgeons are amazing! Over time, this would heal and the bruising would disappear.

ASSISTED SHOWERING

From Day 8 through to Day 12, I was very lucky to have my family members help me with showering. With the left arm bandage removed, I had to protect the arm from getting wet, by using a plastic bag. I also had to make sure that I did not get any water near my neck where the wiring was. Being able to wash my face, lightly brush my teeth and style my hair made me feel great and look more presentable. Feeling fresh and clean set me up for each day of recovery.

DAY 9 AND 10

On Day 9, the salivary secretions finally stopped and equalised. This was a great day and was indeed a big win for me. Deep down I felt that my body was healing and it was a sign that I was getting better. I also had my neck dressing removed. My neck was feeling very tight, but I had more freedom of movement. These two improvements were yet another step of progress in my recovery.

On Day 10, I started my routines of doing physio exercises to improve my neck, arm and shoulder strength and mobility. I also walked up and down the ward and used the massage ball to relieve tensions on my back. I also took lactulose to help me go to the toilet and spent the rest of the time getting some good sleep. Each day there was some improvement. I just had to be patient.

DAY 11 – REMOVAL OF DOPPLER CONNECTIONS AND STITCHING

On Day 11, the doctors gave the okay to remove the Doppler connections. They were very happy with how the flap had healed and were very confident that the vein connecting my neck blood supply to the flap, was no longer at risk. The nurse removed all the blue wiring and dressing from my left shoulder. Then the doctor slowly pulled the silver wiring from my neck. This wire would disconnect from the vein, connected to the flap.

The nurse then meticulously removed the stitches from my neck. These were very fine stitches that were performed by the surgeon to minimise scarring. They did a fantastic job. There was a lot of tweezing and pulling of the stitches, but overall this was bearable. Once they were removed I had no connections, stitches or dressings around my neck. What amazing progress!

The doctors also mentioned that in a few days' time I should be able to start having fluids and foods through my mouth. The first thought that came to mind was drinking coconut water. I just had this urge to drink it, and I could literally taste it and smell it. I really looked forward to this, and yes, I was counting the days.

What drink would you look forward to? Just remember that it has to be non-alcoholic!

DAY 12

The SALT team tested my breathing, tongue movement, facial and mouth expressions, speech and swallowing action. My tongue movement was limited and numb on the left side.

First, I had to get my swallowing reflex tested. This is because over the last 12 days I had not used my throat to eat real food, and had not used my swallowing muscles for that long. The SALT team did a number of tests on me, including giving me a mask to inhale some "citric oxide". As soon as I inhaled this I automatically coughed – this was the response that they were looking for, as this meant that when I ingested food it would not go down into my lung but into my stomach.

As a result, the team were happy and said that they would advise the dieticians that I could start feeding through the mouth. They also said that the NG tube could be removed the next day. That was great news. I told my parents, and asked them to bring some coconut water the following day.

I met up with the dieticians and they advised that I should start after the NG tube was removed. They recommended water, pureed foods only, and also the Ensure TwoCal Milkshakes.

DAY 12 – NUTRITION & EATING THROUGH THE MOUTH

During the morning, the dieticians popped round to see how I was doing, and started me off on drinking a cup of cold water. I sipped it very slowly and could feel it running down my throat into my stomach. It felt great. It was an effort to swallow, as my swallowing muscles were weak, but I managed this successfully. I then proceeded to have some pureed foods, such as pureed fruit. I really enjoyed this. It was very tasty and quite easy to eat.

For lunch I had pureed mash, chicken, and peas, with lots of gravy on the side to lubricate and make it easier to swallow. Sometimes I did find this a bit dry and also found that the food stuck to my tongue. So, after each teaspoon of food, I washed it down with water. I could only have a teaspoon of food at a time as my mouth and tongue could not manage more than this.

I then had a nice yoghurt, which was really easy to eat and very tasty. I was really happy to be eating food again.

That day, after lunch, my parents bought a fresh coconut and emptied the juice into a drink container. They brought it to me during visiting hours, and I remember taking the first sip. Wow! It was so tasty. It really felt amazing to be having something that I really liked.

HISTOLOGY REPORT

The histology report arrived on day 12, in the second week of my stay in hospital. I had been waiting eagerly for this. The consultant advised that they found no cancer in any of the 57 lymph nodes, which were removed from my neck. He expressed that this meant that the cancer had not spread to other parts of the body and was localised. This was fantastic news. I was relieved and happy at the same time. When I think about it, it was a defining moment. My lifespan just got bigger, and I now could focus purely on healing my neck, mouth and tongue.

The consultant then talked about what my next treatment options were. He recommended that I have radiotherapy treatment only. This was based on the histology report and also identifying that the cancer was a lot deeper, during surgery, than was picked up in the MRI and CT scans. They had changed the staging of the cancer from stage 2 to stage 4. Taking this on board, it was advised that radiotherapy would give me the best chance to avoid the cancer coming back. I did think about this for a while, as ideally I didn't want to have any more treatment. However, it was clear to me. I wanted to have peace of mind that I had done everything I could to prevent any recurring cancer. Radiotherapy it was.

The next step was for the consultant to communicate with the oncologist to arrange a series of meetings to explain the treatment details. I had a choice of either Charing Cross or Mount Vernon Cancer Centre to be treated. I took a few days to do my research and went with Mount Vernon. The key reasons for this were: a great reputation for quality of staff, treatment and service, as well as parking, and also I wanted to be away from the city centre and be somewhere more peaceful.

I will talk more about the events that led up to having radiotherapy a bit later in the book, in the chapter titled – Preparing for Radiotherapy.

DAY 13 - SHOWERED BY MYSELF

It is the little things in life that can make you happy. On day 13, I was able to shower by myself for the first time in hospital. This was a great feeling. I'd come a long way since Day 1, it was amazing progress.

DAY 13 - TODAY'S NUTRITION

Here are some of the foods I had on Day 13. You will notice that my appetite had picked up a bit. This was a very good thing.

The Ensure milkshakes and juices would play a large part in my diet in the medium-term, once I left hospital. Here is a photo of what these look like:

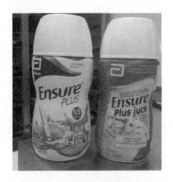

The dieticians highly recommend these, especially if you find it hard to eat enough real foods.

8am:	1 Ensure TwoCal strawberry milkshake.
8.10am:	1 Cup of water.
9am:	Porridge – I found that this stuck to the tongue and so had to rinse this with water.
10.20am:	Pureed fruit – easy to eat.
10.40am:	1 Cup of orange juice.
12 midday:	Tomato soup, pureed Lancashire lamb hotpot, x1 yoghurt, x1 cup of water.
4pm:	1 Vanilla Ensure TwoCal milkshake.
6pm:	Pureed shepherds pie and gravy, peach yoghurt.
7.30pm:	1 Cup of water.
9pm:	Carrot and celery, fresh homemade juice.

DAY 13 - REMOVAL OF THE NG TUBE

After 13 days, the doctors were very happy with the healing of the mouth and gave the okay for me to have the NG tube removed. They also advised that I would most likely be discharged from hospital the following day. This was fantastic news. I felt great, and again I was making progress.

With the doctor recommending that the NG tube could be removed, the nurse helped to remove the tube. I imagined that this would be painful and uncomfortable. I pictured Arnold Schwarzenegger pulling a round metal spherical bomb device through his nose, in the movie Total Recall. Of course, it was nowhere near that bad! Once the NG tube was removed, my throat felt so much better. The irritation and reoccurring cough was no longer there.

DAY 14 – DAY OF DISCHARGE

Day 14 had finally arrived. I woke up thinking, 'This is my last day in hospital. Wow! I have got through so much. Well done.' I had a nice shower to freshen up and spent the rest of the morning writing thank you cards, packing my bag, eating and drinking and then waiting for my family to arrive just after lunch.

I wrote three thank you cards in total. One for all the doctors, surgeons and operating staff that performed surgery on me and supported me through surgery, one for all the nurses that looked after me, and finally one for all the staff at the intensive care unit. During the writing of these cards I felt really grateful and blessed to have such wonderful people there to help me. I actually remembered most of the doctors' and nurses' names, and wrote specific small messages to each of them. If you ever read this, I want to thank you all for your amazing support.

In the Gray Ward they have a wall in the corridor, filled with Thank You cards from past patients. It's great to read those and see so many people that they have helped.

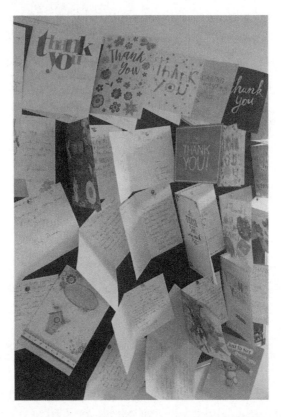

The doctors came to do their morning rounds and confirmed that I was well enough to go home. I gave them their cards and they were all really appreciative and thankful. They advised that the next steps would be to sign some hospital discharge papers, and then I would be okay to leave after lunch.

In terms of medications, the doctors advised that I could either pick up these from the hospital pharmacy before I left, or obtain them from my local pharmacy. I would definitely recommend picking these up at your local, as the hospital one tends to be very busy and you might be waiting a long time.

After lunch, my family had arrived. It was time to go home. I signed the discharge papers and said my thanks and goodbyes to all of the nurses on shift. I also wished all the patients in my bay a wonderful recovery.

Staying in hospital for almost 2 weeks and then leaving these surroundings, was surprisingly great. Getting into the car and watching life outside pass by, on our way home, felt exciting. The fresh air, the different colours and sounds and seeing so many people out and about. I thought to myself, 'I am looking forward to living more life.'

Reaching "home sweet home", I felt very happy and blessed. Walking in through the front door felt amazing and very healing. I had come home.

One challenge was overcome, and now I had to rise to the next one, recovering at home.

CHAPTER 9
RECOVERY AT HOME

Over the next month and a half, I recovered and healed at home. It was the best feeling, being at home. I had my favourite cosy sofa to sit on and watch TV, and of course my own bed. There's nothing like sleeping in your own bed. I felt happy, peaceful and safe being at home with the family.

Getting back my strength and recovering well, was very important to me, as my next challenge would be to prepare myself for radiotherapy treatment. I will discuss this in more detail in the next chapter. In the interim, I will share some of the events and activities I did to get better at home.

LOVELY SURPRISES

Walking into my bedroom, I had a lovely surprise. My parents had the room re-plastered and re-painted. It was an ocean blue colour. I liked it a lot. I found it very calm and tranquil. It was just what I needed in order to help me relax and induce sleep.

If you are reading this because your family member or friend is undergoing treatment for cancer, please know that little surprises are so very much appreciated, and boost morale.

My next-door neighbours were also very nice. They got me a welcome home present, a hamper filled with goodies, which included a new dressing gown, socks and magazines.

Friends of the family would make food and bring it over to the house. This was such a lovely thing to do, as it really helped my family, not having to cook on some days. I can remember having pumpkin soup, prawn and seafood soup and also some amazing Dhal soup. They were all tasty.

Having these lovely surprises definitely boosted my spirits and made me feel cheerful about life. I felt blessed to know that there were special people in my life that really cared.

HOW I WAS FEELING

Over the next few weeks, I looked and felt very tired. But I slept a lot which was great. My body and mind needed this. My mouth also went through a lot of transitions whilst healing:

• My tongue was swollen and I had to be very careful not to bite down on it, as it slightly bridged across my teeth.

To overcome this, I purposely kept my mouth shut with top and bottom teeth touching, rather than apart. I found that helped rather than inadvertently biting the flap.

• My tongue movement and mouth opening was minimal. This meant that my speech was impaired with a lisp on some types of words. There were a number of times where I had to repeat what I was trying to say to others, as they could not understand me.

• I also experienced tingling and burning sensations on the non-operated side of the tongue, over a period of 4 days. I believe this was my tongue healing, with the nerves and feeling coming back to me. I took paracetamol to relieve the pain.

• I also endured lots of coughing throughout the day and especially at night time, when lying down. It was mostly a dry cough.

• I had a slight droop of the bottom left mouth, where the muscles and nerves were impacted by the surgery. This would eventually come back to almost normal, over time.

To improve this, I would massage, under the bottom left lip, and also practice different mouth expressions to improve my mind muscle connection with this area. This definitely helped me in regaining movement and symmetry.

• I had numbness of my face and jaw on the left side.

• I had dry mouth, where there was a lack of saliva being produced. This was one of the side effects of the operation. I made sure I had a bottle of water with me at all times so that I could sip frequently.

• My neck was bruised, swollen and very stiff in movement.

I knew that I had overcome the greatest challenge of getting through the operation and recovering at hospital. Going through the above side effects of surgery, I accepted that it would take time to recover and that I had to take things one day at a time and acknowledge that it would improve each day. Patience was key.

NUTRITION

The food I was eating was all pureed. It had been 2.5 weeks since I had the operation and my tongue had very little movement and my swallowing actions were weak. I needed to build up my swallowing muscles everyday. This was achieved by placing a rolled up towel under my neck and practice swallowing. This was recommended by the SALT team.

I had lots of gravy with each meal, which helped me to swallow smoothly. I also ate with a teaspoon, as my mouth could not manage a lot of food at one time. I ate only on the right side of my mouth, as I was not comfortable or capable of eating on the operated side.

At home, I was very grateful for Mum preparing food for me. One key kitchen utensil was a Handheld Blender. This was very useful in producing pureed foods. Here are some photos of the foods I ate:

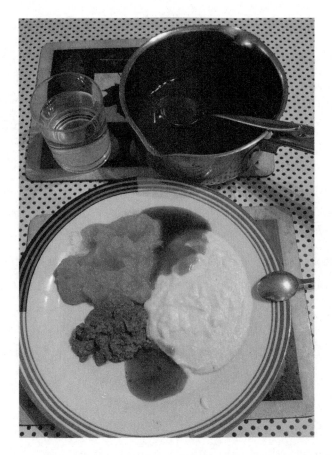

Above you can see the green pureed Broccoli, orange Sweet Potato, white Chicken and lots of gravy. The gravy made eating a lot easier. It was important for me to make sure I ate real, natural healthy foods. I had these at lukewarm temperatures as my mouth was quite sensitive. I also supplemented my diet with 2 to 3 Ensure Milkshakes per day. My dieticians at the hospital prescribed this for me and I had two large crates of this drink available. I was also advised by them to not have citrus or spicy foods, as this would aggravate my mouth.

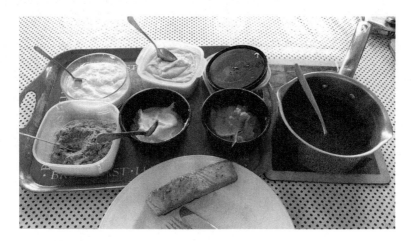

Another meal I had was pureed Sweet Potato, Butternut Squash, and Salmon – this would be broken down into small pieces, white swede, and lots of gravy. A large batch would be made up and I could eat this throughout the day. Having lots of containers to store the food were also important, so I definitely recommend having these.

Four weeks after the operation, I was able to have soft foods with limited tongue movement and mouth opening. During the surgery, they removed part of my salivary glands. This had the effect of making my mouth dry. In order to make eating food easier I found that having 'water-based' foods really helped. I would steam courgettes, asparagus and Bok Choi (the crunchy bits chopped up) so that when I ate them my mouth would feel the juices of the vegetables and thus lubricate my mouth. I also had chopped cucumbers at room temperature. I'd highly recommend trying this out.

TOO MANY BITS

Another thing to note is that having food with too many pieces, e.g. rice, was too difficult to manage. The rice would get stuck inbetween the flap and my teeth and I was unable to manoeuvre my tongue to move the food, and so had to use my fingers.

TOO DRY

Eating dry foods was impossible for me. They were just too dry and were like sawdust. Bread, porridge and biscuits were a no-no, let alone trying one of my favourite foods, pizza.

MOUTH HYGIENE

Throughout the day and after every meal, I would either lightly brush my teeth and tongue and floss, or use alcohol free Corsodyl mouthwash to clean my mouth. I used an electronic toothbrush, which is so much easier to clean your teeth and gums. Definitely get one of these, it makes such a big difference and it is effortless to use. In fact, I looked forward to cleaning my teeth.

CONSTIPATION

With the multitude of painkillers that I had taken at hospital, as well as getting back onto real food, I endured a number of days of severe constipation. It was such an effort to get any movement, that I had to use surgical gloves, to physically assist in this. I simply had to do what was required at the time. Taking Senna laxative tablets, would help to improve things.

In hindsight, I should have tried eating pureed prunes, as I know that this has helped me in the past. I also could have improved my gut flora, as painkillers severely degrade this, by having sauerkraut, kimchi and kefir, yoghurts and of course plenty of water.

DOCTORS CHECKUPS

The week after being discharged from hospital, I had my first checkup, back at Northwick Park Hospital. I was weighed first, by the nurse, which was then recorded in my notes. My weight had dropped from 63.5kg, when first admitted into hospital, to 62kg when I was discharged, and then had remained at 62kg.

I met up with the SALT and Dietician teams, it was great to see them again. They checked my speech and swallowing action, and also asked how I was coping with eating. My swallowing was still quite weak, but I was advised to be patient, as this would improve with time. I was told to try and have more dairy products to help increase my weight. I personally do not like dairy but said I would make an effort to have more yoghurts in my diet. Overall, they were happy with my progress.

It was great to see the doctor who performed the operation on me. He put a smile on my face because I was so very grateful for all he had done for me. He is fairly young with a calm demeanor with a fun and likeable personality. Examining my mouth, he advised that everything was healing as it should and it all looked very well. I had noticed, whilst at home, that there were a few hairs growing from the flap. Whilst this sounded quite strange, it's actually not, as the flap had come from my arm, just below the wrist on the underside. The doctor advised that this was normal and could be removed with laser surgery in the future. However, what I noticed was that these hairs died off when I had radiotherapy.

I also got to meet my oncologist that day. She advised that we would meet up for a full consultation at Mount Vernon Cancer Centre in early November, but prior to that, I would see a dentist to check the health of my teeth and gums. This was in preparation for radiotherapy treatment.

That would be my last doctor's checkup at Northwick Park Hospital until I had completed radiotherapy treatment.

THE MULBERRY CENTRE

I registered at The Mulberry Centre (TMC), which is on the same site as West Middlesex University Hospital, on 19th October 2016, a week after being discharged from hospital. Whilst it was important for me to rest and recover at home, it was just as important to get out of the house and socially interact, learn and have treatments. My mum, who is a retired nurse, knew about this place as she had attended the opening of the centre way back in 2001.

The TMC provided a wealth of free services, for anyone with cancer, from Counselling to Aromatherapy Massage, with many different types of classes, such as Creative Writing and Seated Yoga. They also had coffee mornings where you could meet other people going through cancer. The staff were very friendly and caring.

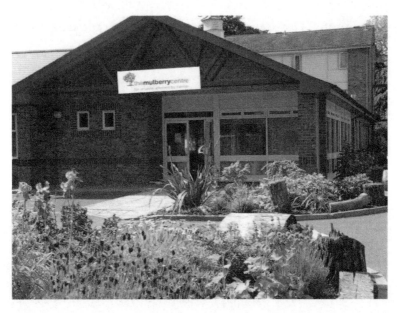

I had a number of Counselling sessions. This was offered to both myself and my mum, separately. We found this very useful and it was great to just talk about things that were on my mind. It is not just the patient that is going through recovery, it is also

Whether you have cancer yourself or are supporting someone who is going through treatment, I highly recommend registering at a Cancer Support Centre near you. They provide a wealth of support and services that will help accelerate your or your family member's recovery.

the immediate family. I am not one for talking to a complete stranger about deep personal feelings, but I remained open to this. I think the open questions helped me to gain clarity on the journey I had been on, and to have an appreciation as to where I was in that moment.

I also signed up to Creative Writing and Seated Yoga classes. I was keen to learn something new which in turn would take my mind away from things. It was also a lot of fun to meet other cancer patients at these classes. By talking and discussing experiences with them, I felt less isolated about my condition and had the realisation that I was not the only one going through this. It was actually quite empowering. Whilst I was recovering physically, I also had to recover emotionally and mentally, so attending these classes really helped.

The Aromatherapy Massages were also a blessing. I had six free treatments and they helped me to relax, soothe me and reduce any tension that my body was feeling.

The Coffee Mornings, every Friday, were a joy. Lots of people would turn up in the morning and it would be great to have a chat. There was a real sense of community and it felt good to be part of something.

DAILY ROUTINES

I am a person that likes to have a daily routine in place. I find it a great way to start my day and add purpose and order in my life. Whilst at home I did the following:

1. Wake up naturally, when I did not have any doctor's appointments that day.

2. Make my bed, brush my teeth, shower, get dressed and have breakfast.

3. Do some guided meditations – I highly recommend trying out *Getting into the Vortex* by Esther and Jerry Hicks. They have a CD that accompanies the book with six meditations. I found these very easy to follow and it helped me get centered, focused, calm and relaxed for my start to the day.

4. Do some journalling which included writing about what I was grateful for and also listing key things I wanted to do that day.

5. I read a lot whilst at home. I had a thirst to find answers within, about how I could heal and make myself better – Physically, Spiritually, Emotionally and Nutritionally. I read lots of books on these subjects.

6. Perform physio exercises, including practising my speech, and tongue, mouth and jaw movements. Sometimes I overstretched my mouth which caused a bit of bleeding near the flap, so I recommend being careful. I also did the physio exercises for my arm and wrist and started using resistance bands for shoulder and back strengthening and stabilising.

7. I exercised outdoors from time to time, walking and jogging in the park. This was a great way to get some fresh air, be out of the house, and work on strengthening the whole body and

getting cardio. I felt so much better after doing this and felt physically stronger for it.

PETS

In March of 2016 my brother had the idea of getting a kitten. We had always been a family that loved cats and felt it was time to get another. The main reason for this decision was so that it would help with my dad's recovery from triple heart bypass surgery. Little did I know, that it would help me immensely in my recovery too.

Having a cat changed the whole feeling and dynamics in our household. The family feels so much love, joy, comfort and happiness with our cat. My cat is called Scooby, he's a lovely black cat and is 2 years old at time of writing.

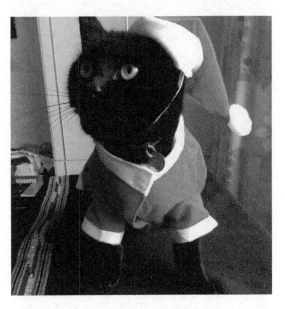

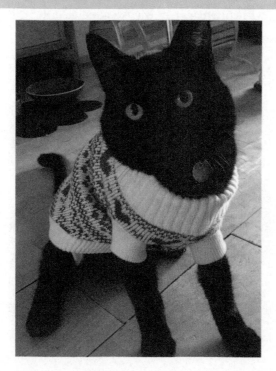

Pets are amazing for post recovery. Cats are quite easy to have, as they are capable of looking after themselves, which makes it easier for you. They make you feel loved and connected and can certainly play an important role in your recovery. You may have a preference for another family pet such as a dog, guinea pig, hamster, rabbit or bird. If you can interact and engage with them, can afford it, and they are not too difficult to manage and look after, then absolutely go for it.

Going through cancer treatments can make you feel very lonely and isolated and too focused inwards with your thoughts. Scooby made me feel more connected and joyful. I forgot about my challenges and was focused on taking care of him. Feeding him, playing hide and seek, grooming and cuddling him. Cats can be affectionate when they want to, especially during feeding time, when he rubs against my leg and meows waiting for his food. This made me feel wonderful inside. Scooby really helped to take my mind off what was going on momentarily and to look forward to how wonderful life could be. Scooby brought a smile to my face.

LAUGHTER

I think it is important to see the lighter side of life and have some fun and laughter. I did this by watching a series called Impractical Jokers. This was a TV show set in America where 4 friends would get each other to do practical jokes on strangers. It was hilarious and made me laugh a lot. If you can find a show or a film that does that for you, then do it. Being cheerful and in good spirits is definitely great for the soul and for your recovery.

FAMILY AND CLOSE FRIENDS

I kept visits to a very few, for my close friends, very good family friends and immediate family. The visits were short so that I did not overexert myself. It felt great to see them all and I really appreciated all their love and support.

PERSONAL RELATIONSHIPS

At the time I did not have a girlfriend, whilst going through my challenges. I found that, with going through major surgery and then being in recovery prior to radiotherapy treatment, I went through a period of "lack of self image". I knew that I was no longer exactly the same and felt that part of me had been removed. Coming to terms with this does take a lot of time and thinking and cannot be rushed. Having your partner be there for you can help you. I was fortunate to have an ex-girlfriend who was there for me. The human connection is a powerful and spiritual force, and it made me feel more normal than I had felt for a while.

WORK AND OCCUPATIONAL HEALTH

The organisation that I worked for were very supportive during my recovery. I have worked for them for 10 years and I was receiving full sick pay for 6 months and then partial pay thereafter. I was very grateful for their financial support. I provided email updates to my Line Manager who in turn would keep my fellow teammates updated. I also started having calls with an Occupational Health consultant, through work, every 4 to 6 weeks. This was to officially record updates on my progress and understand what the next steps were.

My recovery at home was going very well. I was implementing empowering routines and reconnecting socially with others. My family were also doing a lot better and were happy with my progress. This progress was key in having the strength and fortitude to endure 6 weeks of radiotherapy. This was the next challenge ahead.

CHAPTER 10
PREPARING FOR
RADIOTHERAPY
TREATMENT

It was time to prepare for radiotherapy treatment, and in order to make things go as smoothly as possible, I got as organized as I could.

In Appendix A, the 'Timeline of events after hospital', illustrates the key activities leading up to radiotherapy. This will give you a better picture of the timings of preparatory activities, before treatment. I again had to take things one step at a time, in order for me to cope better.

DECIDING WHERE TO GO AND WHO COULD TAKE ME

I chose to have my radiotherapy at Mount Vernon Cancer Centre, because it was highly reputable and it was a dedicated cancer unit. Furthermore, it would be easier to travel by car, outside of London, and there was parking available. The location was in lovely, peaceful place. I was very grateful to have my parents to take me there for my treatments.

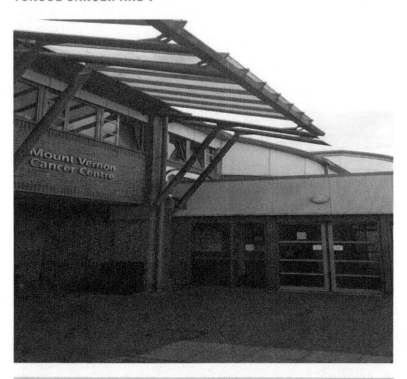

Think about how you are going to get to the hospital every day. What support you will need. The hospital may be able to provide transport services, so do ask. Alternatively, find out if family and friends are available to take you. They can really help here, as when you are going through the side-effects of radiotherapy you do not want to be worried about the journey to and from the hospital.

RESEARCHING RADIOTHERAPY

During my recovery at home, I did a lot of reading about radiotherapy. The Macmillan Cancer Support book, called *Understanding Head And Neck Cancers*, helped me to understand more about it. I recommend reading this, as it explains what the process is, what the short-term side effects are (during treatment and after), and also what the potential long-term side effects are. These are all of the things that I had to weigh up in my mind, and I listed a number of questions to ask, for when I had my consultation with the oncologist.

QUESTIONS:

• Do I really need to have radiotherapy treatment?

• What is the success rate?

• What are the side effects of radiotherapy?

• Is Proton Beam Therapy better?

• Do I need a permanent tattoo, so that the radiotherapy rays can correctly target the cancer area?

• Will I get follow-up scans after treatment?

• Are there any shields that will be used, to prevent reduction in saliva and blood supply to the jawbone?

• What type of external radiation treatment will I have? Is it Intensity Modulated Radiation Therapy (IMRT)?

The answers to some of these questions are covered in the next section.

INITIAL ONCOLOGY CONSULTATION

On the 3rd November 2016, I met with the Consultant Clinical Oncologist, to discuss the treatment plan. It was advised that radiotherapy treatment would be the best course of action for me. This was because during the operation they found that parts of the cancer had spread like tentacles from the main area. These were also removed, but in order to give myself the best chance possible, and kill off any microscopic cancer cells, radiotherapy treatment would be recommended.

I ideally did not want to go through another set of treatments, but realised that I would not have peace of mind if I did not have the radiotherapy. If I didn't take the treatment, I would always be worrying about whether the cancer would come back.

The consultant then explained that the operation to remove the cancer was like pulling the weeds from a garden. The radiotherapy was the weed killer that was spread across the garden (my tongue), to prevent the weeds returning. This really made sense to me, and I pictured the X-rays killing off any cancer cells.

We did discuss a number of the short- and long-term side effects, such as:

- Trismus – restricted mouth opening.

- Xerostomia – dry mouth resulting from reduced or absent saliva flow.

- Dysphagia – difficulty swallowing.

- Osteoradionecrosis – bone death in the jaw.

- Lymphoedema – facial and neck swelling.

- Darkening of the skin around area being treated.

- Tightness of skin

- Mucositis – ulcerated mouth.

- Taste change.

- Excess production of mucus (thick saliva).

- Extreme tiredness.

- Hair loss – facial hair and hair at side and back of head.

I did my research on all of these and it was quite a lot to digest. I decided that I would risk and accept the above side effects, in order to have a longer life. Although many of them risked making my life more challenging, it was far preferable rather than the risk of the cancer coming back. I will talk about what side effects I have now from these treatments, in Chapter 14: Life after Cancer.

The consultant expressed that I would have IMRT. This is external radiation treatment, and was very good in targeting only the areas of cancer and not spreading to other healthy tissue, thus providing better shielding. The consultant then explained the next steps. I would meet with a consultant in Restorative Dentistry, and then meet up again for a radiotherapy planning appointment.

RESTORATIVE DENTISTRY CONSULTATION

On the 9th November 2016, I met with a consultant in Restorative Dentistry. The objective of this meeting was to assess the health of my teeth and gums, and to identify any areas that would be severely impacted by the radiotherapy. For example, if I had any teeth that were decaying, the radiotherapy beams could accelerate this and also impact the gums and nerves below these teeth.

I also had an X-ray taken of my mouth, and the results were very good. I had well-maintained dentition and there was no need for any tooth extraction – I was so pleased with this, as I do try and look after my teeth.

The consultant prescribed GC Tooth Mousse to help with repairing any enamel or dentine, and also Duraphat 5000, which is highly concentrated fluoride toothpaste. Both of these would help keep my teeth and gums healthy and strong, and were to be used during the radiotherapy treatment.

PLANNING RADIOTHERAPY

On the 14th November 2016, I was back at Mount Vernon Cancer Centre. The purpose of the meeting was to have everything required in order for the oncologist and radiologists to plan my radiotherapy treatment. I met up with the radiotherapy support nurse and also the radiographers.

This comprised the following activities:

i.   Taking bloods

ii.   Having a small tattoo

iii.   Creating a mouthpiece

iv.   Creating a face mask

v.   Taking CT Scans

vi.   Providing treatment dates

vii.   Providing medications

viii.   Meeting SALT and Dietetic team

TAKING BLOODS

I first met the nurse who took my bloods. I had not had my bloods checked for approximately 3 weeks, so I guess it was important for the medical team to make sure all was well.

HAVING A SMALL TATTOO

The radiographers gave me a tiny permanent tattooed dot, in the centre of my chest, to ensure that I was in the correct body position each day for treatment. This was a tiny pricking sensation, which was bearable.

CREATING A MOUTHPIECE

The next step was to create a mouthpiece, with an open syringe and plasticine surrounding it. This meant that my tongue was in a fixed position during radiotherapy treatment, and I could breathe through a small pipe airway. The consultant had to mould some plaster into my mouth and I had to let it set for about 5 to 10 minutes. Breathing through my nose made it a bit easier to get through this. Once it was set, the consultant removed it, and this would be sent to the radiographers to keep and then present to me when I first started radiotherapy treatment. It looked liked this:

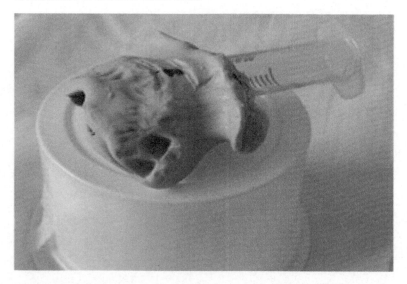

In the above photo, you can see the top view of the mould, where the roof of my mouth would be. You can also see the clear airway pipe, which would allow me to breathe through my mouth.

CREATING A FACE MASK

The creation of a face mask, also called an 'immobilisation shell', was more of a challenge. One consultant asked me to lay down on the CT bed and aligned my head and body correctly. I then placed the mouthpiece in my mouth. Another consultant had a warm green mould (a face mask), which went down to the chest. They placed this over my face and over the mouthpiece. They then started to mould the mask around my face, making sure it was a tight fit, whilst I was breathing through the mouthpiece. This was very challenging, as I felt claustrophobic on the face, but the consultants did well to reassure me, that it would be okay. I tried to control my breathing, breathing slowly from my stomach, and out through my mouth. It worked. I also focused on positive things like silently expressing affirmations, 'This is easy', 'You can do this', and 'It's only for 5 minutes'. I did get through it, but barely. Overcoming it was quite a relief.

The mask looked liked this:

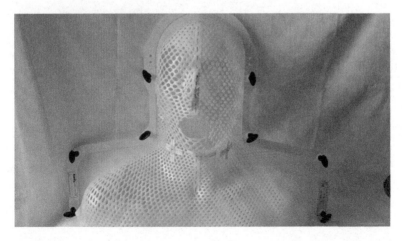

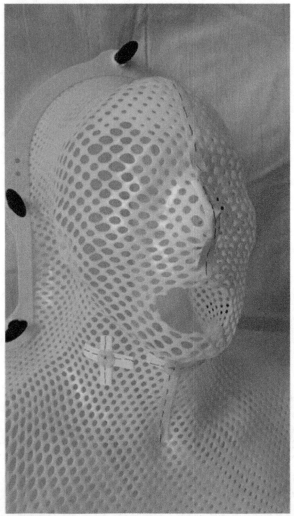

TAKING CT SCANS

I then had to wear the face mask and have a CT Scan (Computerised Tomography). I was injected with a special dye and a number of scans were taken. This was all part of calibrating the line of attack for my radiotherapy treatment.

LIST OF TREATMENT DATES

I met up with the radiotherapy nurse, who provided me with the timetable for radiotherapy treatment. It was a piece of paper comprising the following details:

Patient Name	Start Date	Staff/Resource(s)
MADHAVAN, DEV (patient no.)	30/11/2016 12:30:00	LA7_2012
MADHAVAN, DEV (patient no.)	01/12/2016 13.10:00	LA7_2012
MADHAVAN, DEV (patient no.)	02/12/2016 12:45:00	LA7_2012
MADHAVAN, DEV (patient no.)	05/12/2016 15:55:00	LA7_2012
MADHAVAN, DEV (patient no.)	06/12/2016 16:20:00	LA7_2012
MADHAVAN, DEV (patient no.)	07/12/2016 16:00:00	LA7_2012
MADHAVAN, DEV (patient no.)	08/12/2016 16:30:00	LA7_2012

The above table shows the date and time of treatment, and the third column shows the treatment room location. I was having a treatment every day, except on the weekend, for 6 weeks, which totalled 30 radiotherapy sessions. I have only shown 7 treatments above, to illustrate the information. One thing I did make a note of was the end date for treatment, 10th January 2017, so I knew what I had to work towards.

PROVIDING MEDICATIONS

The nurse also prescribed the following medication and advice on how to take them.

• Effervescent Paracetamol 500mg, to help with pain relief.

• Dispersible aspirin tablets 300mg, and Strawberry Mucilage – to help with pain relief in the mouth, making it easier to eat food.

• Capasol – to prevent ulcers appearing.

• Tellodont 'Gargle and Mouthwash Tablets' – helps to loosen mucus and refresh my mouth.

In the next chapter, I will discuss the mouth hygiene routines put into place when using these medications.

MEETING THE SALT AND DIETETICS TEAM

I also met up with the SALT and Dietetics team. The SALT team would be monitoring my speech and swallowing during radiotherapy treatment. The Dietetics team would advise on and monitor my nutrition. This was important, as I needed to maintain my weight throughout treatment, especially around the face, so that the face mask remained a good fit, as well as helping me to remain healthy and strong.

All the preparations were in place, and I was now ready to start radiotherapy.

CHAPTER 11
HAVING RADIOTHERAPY

Overcoming major surgery and then having 2 months to recover, before having radiotherapy, was another big challenge to embrace and overcome. I will talk about the routines and events that transpired, and how I felt during the 6 week course of treatment. I will also highlight the positive actions I took to endure and surpass the obstacles I faced.

FIRST DAY OF TREATMENT

Wednesday 30th November 2016, the first day of radiotherapy treatment, had finally arrived. I had prepared myself for this as much as I could and I was feeling quite strong and healthy.

Travelling to Mount Vernon Cancer Centre, with my parents and brothers, was very important to me. Having that loving support means everything. Although I had prepared for this, lots of things ran through my mind, whilst making my way there. I'd been here before, when I travelled to Northwick

Park Hospital, for major surgery. The fear of the unknown and having to go through another treatment, made it scary. However, I knew that 'I had to have it', in order to have that peace of mind, and to know that I did everything I could to kill off the cancer, and give me the best chance of surviving and living my life.

Driving through Ruislip and Northwood, on route to the hospital, there's a lot of beautiful green landscape to see from the passenger window. I felt a great appreciation for the nature in life and was grateful that I would see this view everyday prior to treatment.

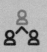

I think the commute to treatments is very important. How you get there and how you feel on the way plays a big part on setting yourself up to be positive, strong, relaxed and grateful about life. A city commute compared to a country commute is quite different, so definitely think about this when choosing hospitals for treatment.

I registered at the reception and was then asked to go to the main waiting area. As I entered, I saw so many people waiting. I was very surprised by the numbers. It must have been at least 40 to 50 people there. Has everyone here got cancer? I wondered. A radiographer then called my name and took me to a waiting room, near where I would have treatment.

In this waiting room, there were at least 15 to 20 patients all waiting to have treatment. Some were being treated for different cancers, some had chemotherapy drips, all in different age groups. Family members, including mine, were there. I said hello to some patients, they gave me a welcome smile, and I smiled back.

While waiting for treatment, I needed to keep myself occupied, as whilst I had a scheduled time slot, these times weren't always met. This could have been due to many reasons, such as unexpected radiotherapy machine maintenance, patient delays etc. On the whole, the radiography team were very good at the set schedule.

I chose to spend my waiting time reading. I read a book called, *The Secret Daily Teachings* by Rhonda Byrne. This is a great book with daily inspiring quotes and teachings. I wanted to prepare for the treatment by reading positive and motivational material. This book is an easy read and helped me to keep strong mentally and also focus on the bigger picture of living my life.

 Find a number of books that you can read which will keep you positive and occupied whilst waiting to have treatment. This will help make you more relaxed, calm and mentally stronger. I chose this instead of flicking through social media, which can paint a lot of different stories, create more noise in your head and make you less focused.

In this particular waiting room they had two treatment rooms. So as two patients completed their treatments, another two patients were called for treatment.

My name was called and I looked at mum and dad, we nodded and smiled, and I then followed the radiographer into the treatment room. There were 3 radiographers who greeted me and they were very friendly. They understood that it was my first day of treatment and they took me through the process, expressing that it would take approximately 5 to 10 minutes to correctly position and calibrate the machine and then approximately 15 to 20 minutes for treatment.

In the treatment room there is the radiotherapy machine with a bed to lay on.

I had to remove all clothing from my torso and I also chose to remove my footwear, so that I could feel more comfortable. I then lay on my back on the bed with my head placed carefully on the headrest provided.

They then gave me the mouthpiece to wear and then proceeded to place the immobilisation mask over my face and upper torso. They then screwed in the mask to the bed so that it was fixed and stable.

The mask was very, very tight on the face and I felt extremely claustrophobic. I was not used to this at all and was very uncomfortable. I raised my right hand and mumbled for them to remove it. They responded in kind. They were very understanding and said to take a moment.

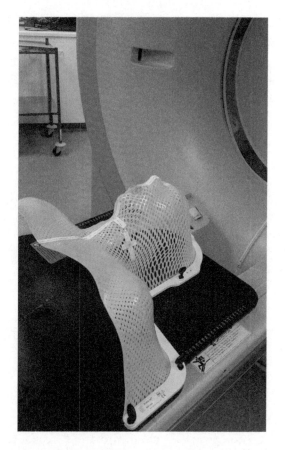

I took a few deep breaths and we retried. But again this was too much for me. I had to stop and take a break. The radiographer said they would ask the oncologist to see if they could give me something to make me more relaxed.

I was then led back to the waiting room. They gave me a tablet, called "Tazipan" to help me relax.

Forty-five minutes later, I was more relaxed and we tried again. This time it was a bit easier. The mouthpiece and mask went on

141

and was secured. The radiographers had a portable CD Player, and played some music in the background.

I managed to block out the tightness of the mask on my face. The radiographers advised that they would now leave the room to start the treatment and would be monitoring from there and talking to me through the speaker.

The radiotherapy machine started to make some noise and the radiotherapy arm rotated around my head. There was a small light that beamed across my chest where they lined up to the tattoo to calibrate and make sure everything was aligned.

They then mentioned over the speaker that they would start treatment.

A 'beaming' noise came from the radiotherapy arm, and I focused on remaining calm.

I breathed slowly into my stomach via my mouth and/or nose, slightly expanding my chest. Then I breathed slowly out through the mouth as my chest and then stomach deflated. Throughout the process, I focused on my breath and had my eyes shut.

I also repeated slowly and silently my affirmations and visualised where I would be after I had fully recovered from treatment. I visualised the amazing person that I am. I pictured me standing tall, smiling in the sun with friends and family around me. I saw a strong, grateful appreciative me, glad to be alive and healthy and feeling so blessed to be with the ones I love. I pictured my amazing niece, and I pictured my brothers and parents, and how proud and grateful I am of them and how I looked forward to spending more time with them.

I managed to get through my first treatment. It was difficult and yes I did struggle. I knew I needed to find a solution that would help me to cope better, because I didn't want to take sedatives every time.

SECOND DAY OF TREATMENT

LISTENING TO BODY SCAN MEDITATIONS

Whilst I was breathing slowly during my first day of treatment, I realised I needed to hear music or something in the room to keep me calm and relaxed.

On day 2, I brought in a CD of guided body scan meditations. This was from the book that I mentioned in an earlier chapter, called, *Mindfulness: A Practical Guide to finding peace in a frantic world,* by Mark Williams and Danny Penman.

The body scans consisted of a calming male voice, which guided me through the meditations. During day 2 I was a bit more relaxed and calm, and I focused on the voice and managed to get through treatment better, without any medication. Having that voice in the room made me feel like I was not alone and also more connected.

Not all treatment rooms had portable CD Players, so playing the meditation CD was not always possible. I managed to get through that day and then took a positive action, to get my own small speaker and attach this to my mp3 player, with the uploaded meditations. I would then play my mp3 player, just before I lay down on the radiotherapy bed and the mask was secured.

The first body scan meditation would take 20 minutes to complete, and this would be approximately when the treatment would finish. This was a good guide for me to monitor and track when the treatment was almost complete. This gave me comfort and reassurance and definitely helped when I had times where I did not think I could continue enduring the treatment, due to being uncomfortable or in a panicked state. The meditation meant I knew how much longer I had to hold on, for the treatment to be completed.

If you are struggling with getting through radiotherapy treatment, try using guided meditations or music via a mp3 player and small speaker.

As well as the guided meditations, there were a few other things I did to make the treatments more bearable.

To improve my breathing, I did the following:

• I made sure that my nose was clear from any mucus so that I could breathe better.

• I also coughed up any mucus from my mouth into a cardboard container prior to going on the radiotherapy bed.

• On some days I would also chew some mint gum or have a mint sweet to clear the airways.

• I had some water just before treatment so that I reduced any feeling of dry mouth.

• I noticed that it was not easy to swallow whilst lying down. Somehow I limited myself from swallowing during treatment. After the first week of treatment, I adapted my breathing. I found that by breathing through my nose instead of the mouth was easier. This was because, when breathing through the mouth, I found that saliva/secretions would build up at the back of my throat during the treatment, and I found it hard to clear these through swallowing.

• I also found that if I pushed my head right to the top of the mask, I was more comfortable. You will need to play around with this to find what works for you. The radiographers helped me get into a better position where my head was as high as it could be in the mask, with the head rest support underneath. This position helped the following areas:

i. I could breathe through my nose - which I found much more easier to do than the mouth - This was major win and made it much better for me

ii. My head was no longer hyper-extended

iii. There was no pressure of the mask on my throat

iv. My shoulders were more relaxed and down

• I got the radiographers to tell me, over the speaker, when we were half way through treatment. This really helped me to relax more. We then took this to another level, by asking them to announce when there was 5 minutes left to go.

• Sometimes there can be problems starting the treatment. I would be lying there and waiting and waiting. I asked the radiography staff to let me know when there were any problems during the treatment and how long I will have to wait on the radiotherapy bed. If I did not hear anything, I would get anxious and there were times like this, where I had to ask the team to remove the mask and let me get up. Communication is key.

I recommend trying these out and I am confident that some of these will help.

After completing the second day of treatment, I felt more confident and relieved that I could manage the treatments, and I felt that this was a breakthrough, and that things would be a lot better the next day. I worked out how to make this work for me.

CALIBRATION EXERCISE

Once a week, the radiographers performed a calibration exercise, taking photos of my mouth to make sure the radiotherapy was hitting the correct spots. This would make the treatment at least 10 minutes longer, so I had to focus on being very calm for this. I could tell that things were longer as my mp3 player would go into the second bodyscan meditation. Again, I focused on the meditation and my breathing, and took comfort in this.

Ask the radiography team to advise when the calibration exercise is. It is better that you are prepared for the longer treatment time.

MONDAY MEETINGS

Every Monday, I was scheduled to meet the nurse, oncologist, a member of the SALT team and a Nutritionist. This would be either before or after my radiotherapy treatment.

In the main waiting area, I would sit with my parents, waiting to be seen. A nurse would call my name and then first lead me to some weighing scales, to weigh me. As mentioned before, it was very important to monitor my weight over the course of radiotherapy treatment, so that the immobilisation mask remained a good fit on my face, neck and shoulders.

The nurse then led me to a room where I would wait for the oncologist to see me. The oncologist performed a general check on how I was feeling and coping with the treatment and made sure I had all the right medications. All was well, as it was my first week of treatment.

I then met up with a SALT Team Member and a Nutritionist. The former checked in to see how my speech was and if I had any issues with swallowing foods or liquids. She also recommended some swallowing and mouth exercises to do, to help improve my speech and movement, as well as exercises to counteract the radiotherapy side effects of jaw and skin stiffness. I will discuss these later in this chapter.

The nutritionist also checked in with me to see how much I was eating. She was keen to make sure I maintained my weight and to also make sure I kept up my strength. She also advised on what to eat and recommended adjustments if something did not agree with me.

It was really great to have such support from all of these wonderful teams.

MOUTH EXERCISES

During radiotherapy, one of the side effects is that the jaw and skin, where the radiotherapy beams pass, can get quite stiff and the jaw opening can decrease. The SALT team member was very keen to monitor this, by using a "Mouth Range of Motion" scale.

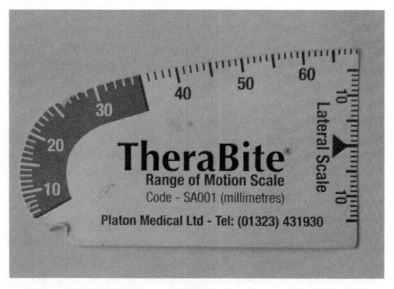

From the diagram, on the left handside, I place the scale inbetween the centre of my bottom teeth (the white part of the scale) and my top teeth (grey part of scale) to measure my jaw opening. My measurement was about 26 millimetres. Our goal was to make sure that this did not decrease, if anything, I should look to improve this. To help me improve this, the SALT team member recommended using Lollipop Sticks bunched together by elastic bands, to stretch the mouth opening, carefully, holding it up to 30 secs.

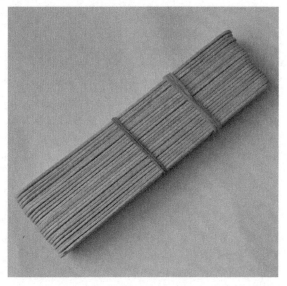

I would do this every other day to keep track of things.

Fast track forward to 2018, and my mouth opening was over 60 millimetres! It's amazing how things progressed.

There were also other recommended exercises that helped with my speech, swallowing strength and jaw opening:

JAW EXERCISES

• Doing an exaggerated yawn and holding this between 5 and 10 seconds. I repeated this a number of times.

• Moving my lower jaw slowly from right to left.

• Doing a chewing action whereby I would chew clockwise 5 times and then repeat anticlockwise, whilst keeping my lips closed.

I found these exercises helped to loosen up the jaw and I could do these anytime. To this day, I still do these exercises.

TONGUE EXERCISES

To help improve the movement and strength of the tongue I did the following exercises:

• Moved my tongue clockwise in circles a number of times and then repeated anticlockwise.

• Moved and pushed my tongue against the inside of my cheeks and then to the top of my mouth and then to the bottom of my lip.

• Stuck my tongue straight out and pushed against my finger and held this for 5 seconds.

SPEECH EXERCISES

• I would practice saying the alphabet and accentuate the words.

• I would practice saying the phonetic alphabet and accentuate the words.

• Place my tongue at the back of my mouth high up, and then say the word hawk. This helped to accentuate the K sound.

SWALLOWING EXERCISES

• Placed a rolled up towel under my neck, and looked downwards, whilst sitting down, I practiced swallowing as hard as I could. Then rested for a bit and then repeated. I found that I could really feel the swallowing motion and realized that my strength of swallowing was weak. I worked on this every other day.

For these exercises, I would highly recommend that you first check with your medical team, before doing any of these.

TRACKING MY PROGRESS

After a few days of treatment, I realized that going through 6 weeks of this felt quite overwhelming. I somehow had to address this. I created my own weekly plan on an A3 Gridded piece of paper, and broke each row into a specific week and then pinned it on my wall to view.

I only had 1 week visible at a time, and then proceeded to tick off 1 day at a time after treatment. The above illustrates what the weekly plan looked like as a whole. This helped me to record the progress I was making. After each week was completed, I would then move the piece of paper over the weekly plan, down by a week, ready for next week's treatment. By breaking things up into a weekly basis, this helped me to overcome feeling overwhelmed by the whole 6 weeks. I chose to focus on one week at a time.

	Sun	Mon	Tues	Wed	Thu	Fri	Sat
WK1				1 ✓ 30/11	2 ✓ 01/12	3 ✓ 02/12	
WK2		4 ✓ 05/12	5 ✓ 06/12	6 ✓ 07/12	7 ✓ 08/12	8 ✓ 09/12	
WK3		9 ✓ 12/12	10 ✓ 13/12	11 ✓ 14/12	12 ✓ 15/12	13 ✓ 16/12	
WK4		14 ✓ 19/12	15 ✓ 20/12	16 ✓ 21/12	17 ✓ 22/12	18 ✓ 23/12	
WK5		19 ✓ 26/12	20 ✓ 27/12	21 ✓ 28/12	22 ✓ 29/12	23 ✓ 30/12	
WK6		24 ✓ 02/01	25 ✓ 03/01	26 ✓ 04/01	27 ✓ 05/01	28 ✓ 06/01	
WK7		29 ✓ 09/01	30 ✓ 10/01				

MOUTH HYGIENE ROUTINE

In the previous chapter, I explained what medications the nurse had prescribed in order for me to manage mouth hygiene and pain throughout the radiotherapy treatment. The nurse did provide a small tick card to keep track of my daily use of medications. However, I decided to create something more comprehensive, which I knew would work for me.

			Wed 30-Nov	Thu 01-Dec	F
		Morning (8 -12)	✓	✓ Physio	
1	Teeth	Brush Teeth with normal tootpaste	✓	✓	
2	Eat	Breakfast	✓	✓	
3	Mouth	Talemon Mouthwash	✓	✓	
4	Mouth	Caphosol	✓	✓	
5	Skin	Aveeno Cream	✓	✓	
		Afternoon (12 -4)	✓	✓	
1	Eat	Lunch	✓	✓	
2	Teeth	Brush Teeth with Fluoride toothpaste	✓	✓	
3	Mouth	Talemon Mouthwash	✓	✓	4pm
4	Mouth	Caphosol	✓	✓	
5	Skin	Aveeno Cream	✓	✓	
6	Teeth	GC Tooth Mouse	✓	✓	
		Evening (4 -8)	✓	✓	
0	Eat	Dinner	✓	✓	
1	Teeth	Brush Teeth with normal tootpaste	✓	✓	
2	Mouth	Talemon Mouthwash	✓	✓	
3	Mouth	Caphosol	✓	✓	
4	Skin	Aveeno Cream	✓		
5	Exercise	Jaw	✓	✓	
6	Exercise	Towel tuck	✓	✓	
7	Exercise	Tongue	✓	✓	
8	Physio	Left Arm	✓	✓	
9	Physio	Neck	✓	✓	
		Night (8 - 12)	✓		
1	Teeth	Brush Teeth with Fluoride toothpaste	✓		
2	Mouth	Talemon Mouthwash	✓		
3	Mouth	Caphosol	✓		
4	Skin	Aveeno Cream	✓		

I created the spreadsheet above, from my first day of radiotherapy treatment, 30th November 2016, to my end date of 10th January 2017. In the above diagram I have shown you 2 days as an example. This spreadsheet helped me to monitor and track when I took the medications. You will notice that I split the day into four 4 hour chunks. I would tick off the printed spreadsheet after taking the medication. I also included the mouth exercises and skin regimes. You can see that I applied cream 4 times a day to my neck and jaw line where I was having radiotherapy targeted. It was difficult to fit this in between meals so I chose to break this up to make it more manageable. You can see how much activity goes into each day outside of the radiotherapy treatments.

MIDDLE OF TREATMENT

In the 4th week of treatment, I started to really feel a bit of discomfort. I developed Mucositis, which are small, tiny ulcers on the inside of my mouth. They were quite sore and sensitive and made it more difficult to eat. To overcome this I would have Soluble Paracetmol 30 minutes before a meal and then 5 to 10 minutes before I would rinse with a Strawberry Mucilage Gel. Both of these really helped to numb the discomfort, so that I could eat.

I also noticed that the taste in my mouth was more metallic. It was not a nice taste. This created a loss of appetite. However, I knew I had to eat to maintain my weight and strength. So I focused on what I knew the foods tasted like which made things a little better, whilst eating.

AT HOME

Throughout radiotherapy I was constantly feeding myself positive information. I would read self-development books every day with positive messages to keep me in a strong and motivated state of mind.

I would also sleep and rest a lot, as I found that the radiotherapy side effect of tiredness, did take a lot out of me. Anytime I felt tired, I would sleep.

I was very fortunate to have my mum cook all my meals, except for me having the Ensure milkshake drinks. This gave me lots of time to rest and not having to worry about preparing meals. I would have at least 2 Ensure milkshakes a day, increasing to 3 on some days. I was eating a range of foods, including scrambled eggs, fish, mashed up sweet potato, pureed broccoli, and yoghurts. I also ate a lot of natural cooked soups like three mushroom (chestnut, shitake and button), butternut squash and carrot soup. These were prepared with lots of garlic, onions and ginger.

I was also keeping in touch with my manager at work, via email, and also the Occupational Therapist, via phone. I would check in every 4 to 6 weeks, so that they both were kept up to date with my progress.

In terms of keeping in touch with family and friends, I chose to not have anyone visit me. Instead I kept minimal contact on social media, so that I could remain focused. It was indeed a busy day, every day for 6 weeks, for both myself and the immediate family. We stuck to a daily routine, getting up early and having breakfast, travelling to the hospital, having treatment, travelling home, eat and then resting before repeating it all the next day. Before we knew it, we had reached the final week.

LAST DAY OF TREATMENT

Tuesday 10th January 2017 was the last day of treatment. I could not believe that I had finally come to the end. The radiography team all knew it was my last day as I walked in with a big smile. They were also smiling. The treatment went smoothly, and as I rose from the radiotherapy bed, I gave a fist pump and shouted, "Yes!". It was a massive achievement to get through these treatments. I then met up with my parents and said, "We did it!". They smiled and were really happy.

I had written out a number of Thank You cards to all the wonderful staff.

I gave a card to the Radiography team and thanked them so much for their amazing support. They had been so patient and understanding.

I also gave Thank You cards to the SALT and Nutritionist team, Reception Staff, Nurses and Oncologists. They were all very happy for me and really appreciated the cards.

As we departed the hospital grounds, I had a big celebratory smile on my face. Six weeks had passed and I had overcome yet another challenge. It had been a team effort. I could not have got that far without the expertise and support from the medical team and the loving care from my family. I am truly grateful to all of them. As this chapter closed, I was now ready to start my recovery from radiotherapy.

CHAPTER 12
RECOVERING FROM
RADIOTHERAPY

I had now completed all surgical treatments for Stage 4 Tongue Cancer, both major surgery and radiotherapy. I was very proud of myself, for having the inner strength and endurance, to get this far.

Now it was time to recover from radiotherapy. My body and mind had taken a battering over the past 3 months, and I knew it was time for more rest and recovery, but also it was time to build myself up and get my life back on track. I will discuss all the activities and alternative treatments I did, from January 2017 to June 2017, to help with my recovery.

SO HOW WAS I DOING?

Every morning, I noticed that my neck was very tight, but then it would eventually loosen up during the day. I would do my neck and jaw exercises to help with this. I also noticed that I'd have dry mouth throughout the day and at night, so would have a bottle of water with me at all times. There are dry mouth sprays that you can buy, as an alternative, but I preferred sticking to water.

On a more positive note, my range of mouth opening and movement had gradually improved, which also helped with improving my speech. I did find that my swallowing motion was fairly difficult, and required focus and effort.

My mouth was also highly sensitive, so I could not eat any spicy food. It had now been almost four months since my last curry.

I would say that overall I was doing pretty well. I had great family support, a roof over my head, food and water, and my health was improving. I was making progress and adapting to the side effects I experienced. There were times when it was a little irritating and frustrating that these effects were so apparent, but I knew that I had to be patient and take it one day at a time.

REST

I spent a lot of time sleeping, taking regular naps, and really listening to my body and mind, which was telling me when to rest. I was very aware of how my energies would fluctuate through the day, so it was important to rest whenever my energy levels were low. This was due to the side effects of radiotherapy and my body healing itself.

THE MULBERRY CENTRE (TMC)

I continued to use the wonderful services at the TMC. I was having aromatherapy massages, attending Friday coffee mornings and attending an 8-week Mindfulness course. This course taught me more about awareness of what I was feeling, being more present in the moment, and being more grounded and centred. This was a great class, as I love learning new things. It was also great because I got to meet other people on their cancer journeys, and it gave me the opportunity to socially interact, which was healthy for my wellbeing.

 As mentioned earlier in the book, post-surgery, I advise finding a cancer support centre. It is also good to return to the centre after radiotherapy, so that you can venture out of the house, remain socially active, learn and achieve new things, and overall improve one's spirits, which is all part of your recovery.

REGULAR CHECKUPS

Every 4 weeks, I would go to Northwick Park Hospital for my checkups. This would be a physical examination and general chat with the oncologist, Macmillan Nurses and doctor, to see how I was doing. It was also an opportunity for me to talk about any issues that I had, which helped me to have peace of mind. I'd also see the Dieticians and SALT team periodically, to check in on my nutrition intake, to see whether or not I needed another batch of Ensure Milkshakes, and how my speech and swallowing were progressing.

WEIGHT LOSS AND NUTRITION

Over the course of recovery from radiotherapy, my weight had decreased from 58.5kg to 55.6kg, from January 10th 2017 (last day of radiotherapy) to June 11th 2017. That's approximately a 3kg decrease over 5 months.

My weight before the major surgery was 63.5kg (October 2016), so 9 months later, I had dropped by approximately 8kg.

Most of my clothes were baggy. My waist size had reduced from 31.5in to 28in, my T-shirt size had reduced from medium to extra small. My tight-fitted shirts now looked like regular fit.

I could see the loss of weight in my face. The rounded healthy shape was more gaunt, chiseled, but overall less healthy-looking. I was going through a very challenging time, in recovering, healing and eating. Though I accepted where I was, there were times when I may have felt a bit down, frustrated and unhappy. However, I chose to not be too hard on myself and decided to look forward. I realised that it would be small steps of progress over a long period of time, that some days I would feel high and others days I would feel low. Nevertheless, I accepted this and cultivated patience and understanding, which helped keep me mentally calm.

Whilst my body was recovering and healing, I believe it was using up a lot more calories, as part of this process. However, my food intake was not enough to accommodate this. I had gotten used to eating less, and was finding it difficult to eat throughout the day. I was also not having big enough food portions at each sitting. The Ensure milkshakes were a lifesaver, as sometimes I just did not want to eat food. To make up for this, I would have two shakes a day.

My mouth was recovering from the mini ulcers caused by radiotherapy. It was mostly discomfort rather than pain. I was still eating pureed foods, but had also progressed to semi-solids. My intake of food was also progressively increasing, but needed to increase a lot more. At night, I found that my mouth was very dry, and I had to take sips of water throughout the night. The disrupted sleep pattern would also have meant I was burning more calories, which was another cause of the weight loss.

The mouth ulcers eventually dissipated a month or two after my last treatment. I also noticed that my taste started to improve. I was also more active from February through to June, so I was burning more calories than I was taking in.

1. Once a week, weigh yourself, so that you can monitor and track your weight. This will help gauge whether you need to eat more.

2. Have regular-sized meals, spaced every 3 hours or so, and if you can track the daily amount of calories, that would help with maintaining and/or increasing your weight.

3. With the double combo of the body recovering and healing plus my increase in activity, I needed to increase my food intake. So I recommend being more aware of your activity levels so that your nutritional intake reflects this.

THE FLAP

The Flap is its own living thing, with its own blood supply from the neck. I found that periodically the top layer of skin on the flap, would shed and a new lighter coloured layer would appear. It kind of makes sense, as this is actually skin from my arm, which is now in my mouth. I also noticed that sometimes the flap would be very firm and other times less so. So I was adapting and getting used to the fluctuations of this.

FULL BLOOD TEST

In March 2017, I noticed that every time I stood up, from a seated position, that I was feeling a bit dizzy and light headed. I saw my GP and was advised that this sounded like Postural Hypotension, and was recommended to have a full blood test. The results of the test were all in the normal range. Eventually this condition passed. It was great to see that my bloods were healthy and I think it is good to get a full blood test every 6 months, so that you can monitor your health.

DENTAL HYGIENE

It was very important for me to have excellent dental hygiene, post radiotherapy. I saw my local dentist for a checkup. This was performed very slowly and gently, as my mouth was very sensitive. Visually, there were no cavities and the gum depth checks would require a few more appointments to assess, as this was painful. I was prescribed a gel and Interdental Brushes to floss with, to help improve the tightness of the gums around the teeth. As part of my hygiene, I brushed and flossed my teeth after every meal. I still continue to practice this today.

SKIN CARE

I continued using Aveeno Cream on a daily basis to moisturize my neck and jaw line, as the radiotherapy had tightened the skin. So this really helped to make the skin feel more soft and supple. The nurses also advised to use Sunblock factor 50, whenever I went outside. The radiotherapy had darkened and slightly burnt the skin, which made it more sensitive to the sunlight. I applied the suncream and also wore a light scarf, for extra protection.

DAILY MEDITATIONS AND READING

I had a daily routine of meditating and reading. My goal was to start my day very slowly, getting calm and centred and really being present with how I was feeling in that moment.

This practice set my day up really well. I felt relaxed and clear minded. During the day, I also read mostly self-help books, to continue my journey of inner work and growth. What I found, by doing these activities, was that I was not focusing all the time on my condition, but instead nourishing myself with empowering activities and living life with purpose.

LIGHT EXERCISE

I began doing some light exercise every other day. This comprised walks in the park, light cardio and weights in the gym, and seated yoga at TMC. I was fairly weak, and wanted to slowly build up my strength. Whilst at the gym, I would bump into people that knew me, and they would say, "Wow, Dave, you've lost a lot of weight". This became a regular occurrence, both inside and outside the gym, and in turn I would say, "Yes, I am working on this, thanks, give me 6 months". I was not ready to disclose what I had been through. I felt like I wanted to first increase my weight and look healthier, and be in a better place, before sharing that I had overcome cancer.

DANCE CLASSES

In March 2017, I felt ready in myself to start doing some dance classes. I was still slightly frail and quite below my normal weight, but I knew that dancing would be great for my soul. This was one of the activities I wrote down in my journal prior to the operation, which I visualized doing in the future.

I had attended many dance classes in the past, and I knew how it made me feel. It brings lots of fun, joy and happiness and my body would feel exhilarated, as if every cell felt alive and were dancing with joy.

I knew this would nourish my soul.

So I went onto the internet and did a search for dance classes in my area and out popped "Lindy Hop" classes. I had not heard of this dance so I watched a video of it. It was amazing, with music from the 1940s and 1950s.

I attended a dance class with a friend and had so much fun. I was hooked and went to a class every week. It was fantastic exercise which brought lots of fun, joy and laughter, and it was great to socially interact with others.

 Even if you are not a dancer, I would recommend trying a dance class. Maybe something where you like the music. Or perhaps an activity which invites you to perform some type of "movement", where you can fully express your body, in some shape or form. It will make you feel better, more energized and uplifted.

UPW CREWING

At the end of April 2017, I volunteered to be a crew member, as part of the Medical Team, at the personal development event called Unleash The Power Within by Tony Robbins. It was a fantastic experience to be part of a team, to support and help all attendees. I had planned and prepared for this by going on

The St. John's Ambulance First Aid At Work Course, in the beginning of April 2017, and qualified as a first aider.

During the event, I had a major breakthrough during one of the interventions about Gratitude. There was some inspirational music playing, while 10,000 people were all standing up in the room. We were asked, "What are you grateful for?" In that moment, I was really grateful to have made it this far, overcoming the challenges that having cancer had presented. I was grateful to be part of life and was really appreciating my second shot. The energy in the room was amazing and I then had a lump in my throat, which led to a natural flow of tears. I made no sound, but just recognised what my body was doing – it was such a natural emotional release. It was so powerful. In that moment, I knew that I was having a breakthrough.

I felt like my body was weeping and healing at the same time. In a way, I felt renewed, like a new chapter in my life was now starting. I hugged a fellow crew member, for a good minute, and began to smile with tears of joy. I felt like there had been a big weight removed from me and I was very happy, peaceful and felt very connected to everything. This brought me back to when I was lying in the recovery ward and also in the general ward, when I almost broke down, but chose not to, as I believed it would not serve me then, but knew that it would happen later in my journey. That time was now and it felt right, to display these emotions and share them with other people.

The celebration of gratitude was such a profound and empowering experience. I called my mum up that day and told her what had happened. I wanted to let her know, as I knew she would be very happy to hear this news and that it might remove some of the weight she had felt.

You may have a similar emotional breakthrough during your journey. It may happen earlier or later and may even happen more than once. But once you have experienced it, you will know, and you will feel more connected to yourself than you have for a while.

PERSONAL DEVELOPMENT SEMINARS

I attended two other personal development workshops across April and May, which were each over two days. This really helped me to keep my mind stimulated and engaged, and to learn and grow, and to get out of the house. It also gave me the opportunity to immerse myself and interact with other people, who value the same thing, learning and growing. The subject matter was on creating a new vision for yourself and creating new goals in your life. I found this quite pertinent, as I was reassessing my future, and it was these seminars that encouraged me to write this book to help others.

BEING SOCIAL

In May, I took positive steps to get back out socially. I attended a number of events that my friends had organised, and I also started dating again. It was indeed fun to be social and meet up with everyone and have some laughs. This was all part of my recovery, getting comfortable being visible again. Being comfortable with who I was now, acknowledging and accepting, that yes, I may be underweight and not fully healthy, but this was okay. I also recognised that my speech may not have been perfect, and that it was a work in progress. So my inner dialogue sometimes may have been critical and judgmental, but again I told myself, that I need to practice and it would improve. During these social gatherings I made a conscious choice not to have alcohol. I was not ready to take this step yet.

BACK AT WORK

In April 2017, four months after radiotherapy, I started back at work, with an 8-week work transition plan, working with the Occupational Therapist and my Line Manager. This plan started with a small number of working hours per week, gradually building up over the 8 weeks. I was very grateful to slowly build up to full-time working again, and had regular catchups to check in on how I was doing.

It had been 8 months since I was last working at full capacity. Most of the work I do is on a computer and involves managing IT Projects. This comprises lots of planning, organizing, prioritizing, monitoring tasks, and involves chairing and attending meetings, with lots of spreadsheet activities. When I started working at this level, my body responded. My body was telling me that this was not normal. I had a skin outbreak. I took swift action and saw a dermatologist privately, who prescribed a steroid cream. This worked really well. The diagnosis was stress from what I had been through over the past year. I put it down to my body adjusting back to work. Eventually the skin outbreak disappeared. My body had grown stronger and could now manage this layer of stress in adjusting back to work.

It was strange being back at work. I appreciated having a daily routine and purpose in place, and it was also nice to work with other people. I made sure that I took things slowly and steadily. However, I did notice a conflict with myself, with regards to the type of work that I was doing. After overcoming cancer, I questioned myself more on how I spent my time and whether or not it was contributing to the world, and making a positive impact on others. I think it is natural to feel this way, as your perspectives on life change. I'll talk more about this in Chapter 14: Life After Cancer.

TENNIS

Tennis has to be probably the best sport in the world. I've been playing this sport for over 35 years and I love it. It was now five months after radiotherapy, May 2017, and I was now healthy enough to get back on the courts and hit some balls. Whilst I was underweight and quite weak in strength, I bought some lightweight tennis racquets to get me started. Building myself up slowly and not over doing it, I gradually improved and began to play tennis at the advanced level that I used to play. Being able to do what you are immensely passionate about, is the best, and it was one of the best things for my recovery. Also, doing things that you used to do, prior to the operation, is a great feeling to identify who you used to be and who you are right now, and it helps to make you feel more normal again.

If you have a sport or activity that you used to do - do it, health permitting. Take your time and be happy with small steps of progress, as it all adds up to your recovery.

CHAPTER 13
TREATMENTS TO AID
RECOVERY

Recovery was a whole new chapter in my life, and with this in mind, I decided to have a number of different treatments, some of them by the NHS and some of them privately. By looking at my health from all angles, this would help me understand where I was in terms of my health, what areas I needed help with or to improve on. It also gave me peace of mind, as I was taking positive steps to move forward and get better.

MUSCULOSKELETAL PHYSIOTHERAPY

On 15th February 2017, I was referred by my doctor, to have physio treatment, at West Middlesex University Hospital, Therapy Centre. This was to undertake a physical assessment to determine what course of action to take to address a slight left shoulder forward rotation and weak supportive back muscles. These were post-surgery side effects that I wanted to reduce, and to help strengthen those areas and improve their function, symmetry and posture.

The physio recommended a number of strengthening exercises, using resistance bands, all of which could be performed at home. Some of the key exercises included external rotator cuff movements, seated pulls and straight-arm pull downs. When I tried these exercises, I struggled and could feel my left stabilizer back muscles shaking. I knew I had a lot of work to do.

The physio also recommended a number of arm movements and core exercises. One of these was called The Bird Dog and was particularly challenging. This involved being on all fours and then pointing straight out the opposite arm and leg, whilst maintaining a strong core. I could not do this exercise. My left stabilizer back muscles were not strong enough. Even when I stayed on all fours and tried pointing my left arm straight out, I could not do this. This was okay, I knew I had to improve in this area and that it would take patience, focus and practice.

Definitely see a physio if you have weaknesses in the areas described. I eventually could do these exercises after 3 to 6 weeks.

MYOFASCIAL RELEASE MASSAGE

In March, my brother recommended a sports massage therapist that also specialised in Myofascial Release Massage and also Therapeutic Massage. I had not heard of this type of massage before and immediately booked an appointment.

I had a lot of tightness along the neck, from the scarring of the neck dissection, plus scar tissue under the jaw line. My objective was to see if this could be loosened and provide more comfort, which could also in turn improve my swallowing reflex.

The therapist analysed my posture and immediately saw that the left side of my neck and the connective tissue was pulling and bringing my left shoulder up and forward. She also identified the tightness of the scar tissue directly under my jaw line.

For the next 8 months, I would see the therapist approximately once or twice a month to help loosen up these areas. This treatment really helped a lot, and I continue to have this treatment periodically, to this present day. I definitely noticed the improvement in movement around the neck and jaw line, and this also improved the movement of my mouth and my speech. I especially felt the benefits immediately after the treatment. The neck area felt much more relaxed and loose, without the tension that I had gotten used to.

I definitely feel that these treatments should be provided to patients, as I strongly believe it would greatly benefit their recovery. I would also recommend investigating "ScarWork" treatment. This is something that I have not tried yet, but again I was told to look into this. It helps to reconfigure the soft tissue and reduce the adhesions of scarring. It does have similarities to Myofascial treatments, but specializes on scars.

CHIROKINETIC THERAPY (CKT)

A very good friend of mine recommended trying Holistic therapy, as another way of seeing how I was recovering. I had a number of CKT treatments, both in person and remotely. CKT is a non-invasive kinesiology technique, which uses muscle testing, as a way of determining and correcting any imbalances within the body, by redirecting energy to depleted areas.

I was keen to see if I had any energy blockages, structural imbalances and how my immune system was doing, and to see if harmony and balance could be restored. The practitioner implemented a number of hand movements and flicks over the head and body, as well moving the patient's hand and arm, asking questions, which provide responses of yes or no, based on the flex and looseness of movement.

The practitioner identified that my throat chakra was imbalanced, and proceeded to redirect healing energy via my cranial energy portals, to restore balance, and break that negative cellular memory. I felt indifferent during the treatment. It was also identified that I was healing very well overall and that my cells were strong.

CKT not only addresses the physical, but also looks at the emotional and spiritual health. The practitioner identified that 4 to 5 years previously, in 2012/2013, I had a strong emotion of fear, which caused an imbalance in my life. This may or may not have been a prime cause for my cancer, but it is something that required consideration. This was actually a period where there were a number of family bereavements, which was a very tough time for the family and I. At the time of this treatment, I did not realise that this could be the cause of emotional fear in the body, and this was not something that could be released so easily. So, I am still working on this, implementing practices of forgiveness and working with a CKT practitioner.

After all CKT treatments, I felt that I had more clarity on some of the effects that past events had caused, and it helped me to release these and let them go. I also had more insight to my health by addressing it from another perspective. This gave me peace of mind and I felt that this was improving my recovery.

SCENAR THERAPY

In early June 2017, I had two days of Scenar Therapy. Scenar stands for, "Self-Controlled Energo-Neuro Adaptive Regulation". It is a hand held device, which sends an electrical impulse through the skin, to the brain; to help the brain release neuropeptides and pain relieve mechanisms. Many athletes have used this to recover from pain and inflammation.

I was recommended this treatment from another therapist, as I wanted to reduce the numbness, improve the symmetry and movement, and get more feeling, on the left-hand side of my mouth and jawline, and restimulate the nerves there, from the side effects of surgery. The doctors do say that there might be nerve damage after surgery, but I wanted to have peace of mind, and see what this treatment could do.

The Scenar consultant passed different levels of electrical current through the device, and brushed it over my mouth, jawline and neck areas. I felt a tingly and pulsating sensation on my skin, and it felt like it was doing good. It was soothing and relaxing and treatments could take up to 45 minutes.

The consultant expressed that sometimes surgery could get in the way of the body's natural healing process, so Scenar helps to re-establish this healing mechanism. After the treatments, I was advised that there was no permanent nerve damage, based on the consultant's opinion, and that the body took to the treatment very well. Over the coming weeks, I believed that this treatment did help me have a better connection and feeling on my left hand side of the mouth. This treatment may not be for everybody, but if you are open to it, I would recommend doing your own research, and consider this as an option to help you in your recovery.

By July 2017, I had made a great recovery. I was now working full-time, playing a good level of tennis and also socially active. My health was improving and I was adapting really well to the side effects of surgery and radiotherapy. I felt good in myself. I could now do the things that I loved and share wonderful experiences with family and friends. I also had a new perspective on life, realising that life is just too short and that you never know what you will be challenged with next. So it became very important to me, in how I chose to live and value each day. I was now ready for the next chapter, Life After Cancer.

CHAPTER 14
LIFE AFTER CANCER

I want to thank you, honour you and appreciate you, for your time, energy and courage in reading this book. Thank you for going on this journey with me. Belief, Hope, Self Discipline, Patience, Acceptance, Resilience and Taking Action, are some of the key qualities that got me through this. These qualities, in conjunction with the wealth of support from the NHS, family and friends, made the path to healing and recovery a lot more achievable.

There are so many things to look forward to after cancer. I want to share some of these with you and also talk about how I am doing.

Life after Cancer, what does this actually mean? To me, it means that I have successfully recovered from cancer and I am living life, being able to do what I like and love to do. To accept any side effects and limitations of surgery and radiotherapy, and embrace life. Yes, I may have lost some stuff, but I have also gained so much too.

SO HOW AM I DOING?

Overall, I have improved over the years. I am looking much healthier and also eating much better. I also have more confidence in myself and am in a happier place. I do still have some lingering side effects, which I will come onto now.

NECK

My neck still has a stiffness where the scar tissue remains, from the neck dissection. The scar has healed up really well, as shown below:

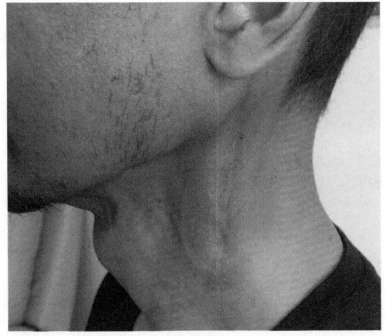

I continue to do jaw exercises and stretches to help with the tightness and also have myofascial massages. I have yet to have scar tissue treatment, which helps to reduce adhesions, so this is something I intend to pursue.

ARM

The scarring on my arm has also healed up really well.

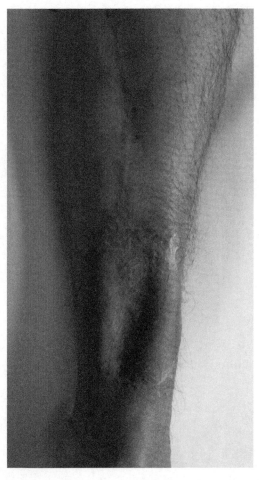

The round part feels like leather but has become softer over time. There is less of a pull on the skin when I flex my thumb.

I am not inhibited in any way. I can snap my fingers, with my thumb and middle finger, easily, which was something I could barely do when recovering at home after surgery. Things definitely do improve over time.

FLAP

I have adapted to the flap really well. It looks very much like part of my tongue with a similar texture and colour. Somedays, it may be hard and tight at the back of the mouth, and other times it feels quite turgid. Then there are moments where I forget that it is even there. I do still, periodically, catch part of the flap on the corner of my teeth, when I am eating. However, I have been more focused on my chewing, to avoid this. Also, sometimes food can get caught inbetween the valley of the flap and gums, where I either have to rinse with a drink or use a finger to dislodge the food for digestion. Overall, I have learnt to live and get comfortable with my flap.

DRY MOUTH

I find I do not need to carry water with me wherever I go now, as my mouth is so much better. Carrying chewing gum will suffice, if required. I rarely get the dry mouth, only sometimes at night.

SWALLOWING ACTION

This has really improved. However, there are some days when

I find it can be quite difficult, but once I do jaw and neck exercises and also swallowing exercises, with a rolled towel under my neck, things improve. I also find that I have to tilt my head slightly forwards to swallow better. I will continue to practise and exercise, until such a time when things feel easier.

SPEECH

I have made improvements in my speech. I have observed, during recordings of myself that I have a tendency now, to make a chapping sound, between long sentences. This I believe is due to the lack of saliva between the flap and teeth, plus the difficulty in swallowing and tightness of the mouth. Whilst this is not highly noticeable by family and friends, it is something that I have noticed in myself. I'd say that I have 95% of the original way I used to speak. I do also sometimes have a lisp and also a lack of pronunciation with some words. With this in mind I continue to practice and record my speech, on video. I find that if I have a slower cadence and pause and swallow silently, between sentences, I speak much better. I'll keep working on this and also remember to appreciate what I do have – that I can indeed speak and others can understand me.

SYMMETRY

Under the left side of my chin and jaw, there is a lot of internal scar tissue. It is very hard and tight, and pulls in conjunction with the scarring from the neck dissection. This causes my left side of chin to be slightly less symmetrical than my right side. It is something that I notice more than others. I think this is because I have a clear imprint on my visible identity. I have taken time to digest and accept these small imperfections. I acknowledge that it could have been worse, so I appreciate what I do have, and continue to exercise and massage these areas to improve movement and lessen the tightness.

TASTE, NUTRITION & WEIGHT

My taste has improved post-radiotherapy recovery. In fact, it is better than it ever was. This might be due to the regeneration of new taste buds. Nevertheless, I now have a greater appreciation for food. My taste is a lot more profound, with wonderful sensations taking me on a journey of discovery and happiness. It is as if I am trying some foods for the first time.

I can now eat most spicy foods, as over time I have been building up the tolerance levels. This means I can eat one of my favourites, Prawn curry with Garlic Naan. My mum, also likes to throw in a few cheeky chillies in some of the meals, without me knowing, which can sometimes make me break into a sweat and end up gulping down some yoghurt, to help calm the palate.

Another one of my favourites is of course pizza. I can now eat this as well.

Overall, I can now eat most things and my love for food has grown.

There are also times, when the mouth might be a little sensitive, where spicy and citrus foods, can be a bit too much, which is okay. However, generally, most of the time things are great.

My diet is mostly a well-balanced healthy one, but this also does include indulging in crisps and chocolates. So, yes mostly healthy organic foods but also the fun snacks too.

As I am eating more, my weight has also increased. I am now 62.4 kg, with a healthy BMI of 21. This has actually taken me 4.7 years, just prior to surgery, to get here. I was originally 63.5 kg, when I went into hospital, so 62.4 kg is not far off from my original weight. Also, during my recovery from radiotherapy, I had reached a lowest weight of 55.5kg, so there have been massive improvements since then. I did not force myself to try and put weigh on, rather, I did this organically and naturally.

It really feels great to eat everything I love and to be at a healthier weight. It is a journey that definitely requires patience, being kind to yourself and taking small steps of progress, at your pace.

HOW AM I LIVING MY LIFE NOW?

I am now more of a go-getter, rather than one that spectates and waits around. I realise that there are no guarantees in life and you have to seize opportunities and enjoy the moments that you have. I now choose not to waste any time. I'd say that I am bolder in life's pursuits, and more purposeful. I have a newfound hunger for growth, applied knowledge and meaningful connections with others. I choose to put myself in positions where I have minimal or no regrets. I continue to fulfil my passions with the things I like and love to do, and embrace each miraculous day with a gratitude, excitement and curiosity. I have a greater sense of awareness, to know when my body and mind is getting stressed or is fatigued in any way. In these instances, I make the conscious choice to slow down, reduce the number of plates I am juggling, and rest and recover.

So, what else have I been up to?

MOUTH CANCER WALK

On the 30th of September 2018, I had the honour and privilege to attend this amazing cancer walk, which was created and organised by The Mouth Cancer Foundation (https://www. mouthcancerwalk.org). Its purpose is to increase the awareness and raise funds, for all head and neck cancers. People from all around the country travel to Hyde Park once a year, to do the 10km walk. It was amazing to see so many cancer survivors, family and friends of cancer survivors, doctors, consultants, nurses, medical staff; all there for this incredible day.

I was greatly honoured and blessed to walk with Dr. Ahmed (on my left in the photo). Dr. Ahmed is my surgeon and performs miracles! When I look at this photo, it brings me great joy and appreciation for this incredible person who helped give me a second opportunity to live a full life. Thank You Dr. Ahmed.

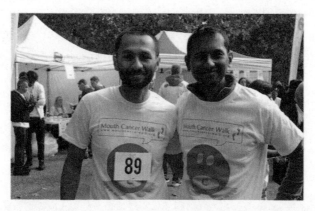

TENNIS COMPETITION

I'd been playing a lot of tennis and was now ready to compete again. I consider myself a club standard player but also enjoy the competition. I competed at a Grade 4 Level at an ITF Seniors Tournament at Rafael Nadal's Academy, in Mallorca. The tournament was on clay, which I am not used to, but I actually loved it. It was so much fun. I managed to get to the semi finals, where I had a tough 2 hour match – a testament to my newfound fitness – which I eventually won. In the final I played the no.1 seed, and gave my best but the opponent was very seasoned on clay and was the better player on the day. It was a great experience and it is great to do the things which you love to do. To play tennis at this level, after my health challenges, was really amazing and shows that there is still so much life after recovering from cancer.

HOLIDAYS

I made the most of my recovery by going on a number of holidays with family and friends. I was wasting no time. I went to Singapore, Malaysia, Bali, and the Dominican Republic and they were really amazing. I also went to New York for the U.S Open Tennis Grand Slam Event and also The Australian Tennis Open in Melbourne; The Laver Cup in Geneva, and of course Wimbledon and the Queens Club Championships. I was so grateful to be travelling again. I do love the sense of adventure, and experiencing something new.

WORK

I have been very fortunate and grateful to remain in work throughout this journey. The organisation that I work for has been very understanding and has helped a lot to adapt my workload, so that I have a better work/life balance and integration. This has really helped me going forward, and really gets the best out of me.

I am now in a place where I can perform at the work capacity that I used to do, however, I have chosen to reel this in, so that I effectively manage my work/life balance and integration. I have also approached my work with a newfound curiosity and interest, looking at how I can make it more fun and enjoyable, more light-hearted but with an intention of adding value, making improvements and delivering results.

GIVING BACK

I am now in a place where I want to help and share more with others.

This is precisely why I have written this book – to help those endure and overcome their cancer journey.

I volunteer and mentor others to find their own paths of awareness and leadership. I also donate to a number of charities, which resonate with my values. Part of this does have something to do with my legacy. I do ask myself, "Have I made a positive impact on others and to this world? This is something you may also wish to ponder and reflect on.

WILL IT COME BACK?

I believe that there are no guarantees, with respect to the cancer being permanently gone and that it might return someday. However, I chose to set myself up to succeed as best I can. The doctors advise, that after 3 years, post radiotherapy, without any further symptoms, it is very unlikely to return. This is fantastic news, as I am approaching 4 years and 7 months, as I write this paragraph. In fact, my next doctors check up will be my last one, as once you reach 5 years post-operation, you are discharged. This is amazing.

I continue to live my life with the following choices, in order to help reduce cancer risk:

• Very rarely drink alcohol

• Do not smoke

• Practice safe intimacy

• Practice regular mouth hygiene, especially after meals

• Practice meditation every other day

• Manage my stress levels very well

• Make sure I rest enough

• I do not rush to do things

• Eat a well balanced diet

• Exercise nearly every other day, both in nature and the gym

• I also get my bloods checked every 6 months, to make sure

my vitamin and mineral levels are on point.

The above is in addition to doing the things I love that feed my soul: Learning, dancing, playing tennis, helping others, and travelling.

I do try to seize each moment of each day and believe that I have to live a life fulfilled with very few regrets.

I am now a lot more time conscious and I do have a bucket list that's growing, with lots of amazing things to look forward to.

LEARNINGS

There are many 'nuggets of gold' that I have included in this book. The majority of which have successfully got me to this happy and healthy place where I can enjoy and live life to its fullest.

Regardless of your situation or where you are in your own journey, I hope you apply some of these learnings and reap the benefits and also share them with others.

HOPE AND COURAGE

We each have our own challenges in life. These test our character, our own belief and hope, and our courage, each day. These challenges give us our inner strength and resilience, to keep moving forwards. External to this, are the bedrocks of strength and support, from our loved ones – family and friends. Challenges improve our ability to adapt to whatever comes our way, and to accept 'what is', which helps us to live each day, and grow in our next best self. I know that I am a better version of myself, after overcoming cancer and I have a deep appreciation for the miracles of life.

LEARNING DURING COVID-19

The lockdowns caused by the COVID-19 pandemic brought a new type of challenge. Being in lockdown, for over the majority of a year, could have been very difficult. I personally chose to see this as an opportunity. Fortune had my back by introducing me to Mindvalley, a world-leading online training platform for Personal Growth. An advert appeared on my Facebook feed, in early March of 2020, for new Health and Fitness training quests. I liked what I saw and signed up immediately. Over the next 7 weeks, I learned and trained each day, to get fitter and healthier. After successfully completing this programme, I was in really good health and shape. I then progressed onto doing other exciting quests, and found that this really helped make the most out of lockdown.

I find that taking an action opens up doors and opportunities, and this was one of them. It helped me to also connect globally with other tribe members, doing these quests. I made new friends in this community, and it made me feel less isolated in lockdown. I created a sense of purpose and direction, and had daily goals and routines, to help me through this period.

CLOSING REMARKS

There is definitely life after cancer. I have a hunger, thirst and curiosity for life. I look forward to each and every day, appreciating all the wonderful things that I have and all the things the world has to offer.

Looking back, it was a tremendous team effort. From my family and friends, to the amazing NHS doctors, surgeons, consultants, oncologists, radiographers, nurses, dieticians, speech and language therapists, physiotherapists, counsellors, The Mulberry Cancer Centre and all its staff, and all of the alternative treatment specialists. They have all been key to my successful recovery. I again would like to say a BIG Thank You to them all, for their dedication to their profession and their amazing and loving support and care.

This team effort made it easier for me to remain mentally strong and have that warm energy of hope and steely-eyed determination and resilience, to keep moving upwards and forwards. Believing and visualising myself doing all the things I love and like to do, until they become true.

I continue on my journey of growth and learning and look forward to what unfolds. Each day is indeed a blessing, and I look forward to seizing every moment.

For those of you that are going through your cancer journeys, I wish you the best and hope this book helps to provide a guiding light of hope, and sets you on a path to recovery. For the family and friends, supporting their loved ones, I hope this book helps you to better understand their challenges, as well as yours, and enables you to serve them and yourselves more lovingly and effectively.

Keep moving forwards and keep improving.

Don't count the days, make the days count.

Muhammad Ali

TIMELINE OF EVENTS IN HOSPITAL

OCTOBER

	MONDAY	TUESDAY	WEDNESDAY	THURSDAY	FRIDAY	SATURDAY	SUNDAY
Date					30th	1st	2nd
Events					Day of Operation — Intensive Care Unit Ward	Started Walking	Moved to Bay A3 General Ward; Catheter Refit; General Ward
Date	3rd	4th	5th	6th	7th	8th	9th
Events	Removal of Drain from Left Upper Leg; Removal of Intravenous Drip and Catheter		Removal of Drain from Chest	Removal of Last Drain from Chest; Moved to Bay C3 in afternoon; Chest X Ray; General Ward	Left Arm Bandage removed; Meet Physio and start neck, arm and shoulder exercises	Tummy Bandage removed; Neck Patching removed; Salivary Excretions Stop and Equalise	Took Lactulose for Constipation
					Excess Salivary Secretions		
Date	10th	11th	12th	13th	14th	15th	16th
Events	Removal of Sponge Dressing on left arm; Removal of Neck Dressing and Stitching; Removal of Doppler connections	Speech Therapist Tests my Swallowing Reflex; Start Drinking and Eating Pureed Foods through the mouth; Histology Report Received; General Ward	Removal of NG Tube	Discharged from Hospital			
		Excess Salivary Secretions					

TIMELINE OF EVENTS AFTER HOSPITAL

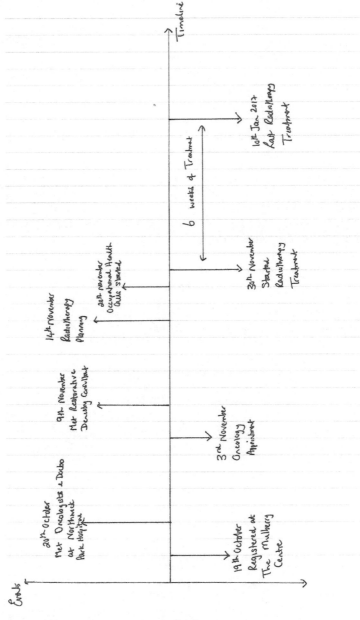

BIBLIOGRAPHY

Mindfulness: A practical guide to finding peace in a frantic world by Mark Williams

Forgive for Good by Dr. Fred Luskin.

Macmillian Cancer Support *Understanding Head And Neck Cancers*

Macmillian Cancer Support *Work and Cancer Guide*

The Secret by Rhonda Byrne.

The Secret Daily Teachings by Rhonda Byrne

The Key to Living the Law of Attraction by Jack Canfield and D.D Watkins.

The Art of Happiness by HH Dalai Lana & Howard C. Cutler.

Aspire by Kevin Hall.

Healing and Recovery by David R. Hawkins

Getting into the Vortex by Esther and Jerry Hicks.

ACKNOWLEDGEMENTS

Whilst the writing of this book has been a solitary and creative experience, there are a number of key contributors that I would like to thank.

The manuscript began in 2016, when my mum, Indra, was my sounding board, and proofread the raw cut version. Thanks, Mum.

My deepest gratitude and thanks to Michelle Gordon, who was so helpful in the production of the book. Thanks for bringing this book to life.

Thank you to all my teachers, healers and creators, both past and present. You continue to inspire and have helped me on this journey.

If this book has been useful, please do consider leaving a review online, and if you would like to give Dev feedback, please email him at tonguecancerandi@outlook.com

Printed by Amazon Italia Logistica S.r.l.
Torrazza Piemonte (TO), Italy

26438103R00120